STOP ALCOHOL FAST:
55 METHODS THAT ACTUALLY WORK
by Gary Pickler

STOP ALCOHOL FAST: 55 METHODS THAT ACTUALLY WORK

by Gary Pickler

Copyright © 2018, Gary Pickler

ISBN13: 978-1-387-87512-2

First Edition   : June 2018

Cover design   : Gary Pickler

Copywriting   : Donna Worden

Editing, proofreading, page design, book design

                            : Bruno Curfs, Gary Pickler

Publisher   : Gary Pickler, through Lulu

Table of Contents

No Stone Has Been Left Unturned Here

I've done my best to approach the issue of stopping alcohol from *every conceivable angle*! There is a very powerful hypnotic method. There are four different depression-stopping methods. Two methods of "getting high in other ways" are included. Four "building super health" methods are here. Several methods of "tripling your willpower" are included. A number of powerful herbs are mentioned that can greatly assist, here. Using lucid dreaming, a Vision Quest, or meeting an inner guide in hypnosis (or your dream) can illuminate your way to stop. Using raging anger to stop, can work. Several methods where your "Drinker" side *finally* talks it out with your "Stop!" side, can effect a solution.

Psychological methods are in here, of getting to the *real* reason why you drink, of crying out your angst, of feeling your nine most-powerful triggering emotions behind all this, of actually learning to truly love yourself instead of drinking, of effectively rewarding yourself for stopping, of using affirmations in ways that *finally work*, of managing your life *far* better in all areas, of enlisting other powerful parts of your psyche to team up with your ego, to quit!

There are unusual methods using ultra-powerful Asiatic hypnosis, banishing rituals, and using stop-alcohol *spells* on yourself. You can "brainwash" yourself to stop, use Mesmer's "Animal Magnetism" or subliminal message to quit, make use of powerful meditation, or even just switch to medical marijuana! You can even boldly face your upcoming death (from alcohol) by walking in graveyards, until you quit!

Several miscellaneous methods, never seen before, are included too.

All-in-all, there are 55 totally different methods here, *all explained fully in detail*. After familiarizing yourself with them all, take your pick! Choose one of the 55 methods that really seems to *fit* you and *your unique style of quitting alcohol*. Then, do it! And then, finally, be alcohol-free, to start living the happy, successful, cured-from-alcohol life that you've always wanted, deep down in your soul!

Why I Wrote This Book For You And Others

I feel enormous compassion for all those struggling with alcohol. It's because of these deep feelings that I want so much to help. My favorite niece, Stephanie, died young from her severe abuse of alcohol. So I'm very motivated to help, however I can, with this book.

Over many decades, I've known several dozen people who miraculously escaped alcohol's clutches. When I questioned them as to *how*, they all freely confided their techniques to me. In this way, I gradually collected *several dozen* methods, over time. Eventually, I knew it was finally time to write this book.

I sincerely hope this book makes a difference with you, and others in the world. May it greatly help all those needing *alcohol-stopping tools*. For not only is this book dedicated to my niece Stephanie, but to all other people in the world who would appreciate *some* help with their alcohol struggle.

From the bottom of my heart, I offer this book to *you*, as a useful tool to help your alcohol issues. May it greatly help you to heal and change your life, so that you'll be happier and more successful.

Even if only *one* person in the world uses this book to more-effectively deal with their alcohol issues, it will be a success.

God Bless!

34 Methods That Stop Alcohol

Method #1 - Gurdjieff-Inspired System of "Weaning"

In a book by Fritz Peters, "Gurdjieff Remembered," pages 50 to 52, the wise but controversial sly rascal/guru figure Gurdjieff, treated a client in a way similar to the following method. To gradually taper off the client's "alcohol over-indulgence," was Gurdjieff's goal.

Gurdjieff advised his client to regard the alcohol consumed daily as "medicine." And, this "alcohol/medicine" needed to be carefully measured out, as it was consumed throughout the day. Thus, every amount of "alcohol/medicine" that the client was about to drink, was carefully measured out (as to quantity), and then this figure was to be entered into a special recording notebook, including the day (and time of day) that it was consumed.

The official medicinal purpose of the "alcohol/medicine" consumed was, of course, to medicinally stop withdrawal symptoms from occurring. Also, to promote the relaxation, stress-reduction, and well-being of the client.

Every day, slightly less "alcohol/medicine" was to be measured out, with each alcohol drink as it was consumed. Thus, the client was gradually getting "weaned" off the daily "alcohol/medicine" consumption by this method! And, the client was relatively free to decide *how much less* was consumed daily, as long as the daily reduction was consistent.

A daily enema, or colonic irrigation, was also performed by the client, to greatly facilitate the toxins from the "alcohol/medicine" more speedily exiting the body. It was considered very important *not* to neglect the daily enema when using this method! So, don't leave out the daily enema, here! (Incidentally, a metal enema hose that attaches to your shower head can be ordered on the internet.)

The reason why the daily alcohol was to be regarded as "medicine," was to *psychologically unify the warring parts of the client*. Then, the unification of the two warring factions in the client, would result in the "unity/willpower" to successfully carry out this method to completion!

See, most overindulging drinkers of alcohol have two sides to their personality. There's "Mister Drinker." And there's also "Mister Stop." Usually Mr. Drinker enjoys the pleasure, fun, adventure, socializing, partying, and "feel-good" effects of alcohol. And often Mr. Stop is upset about alcohol ruining one's health, causing embarrassing drunken incidents, costing too much, and (in general) wrecking one's life!

Mr. Drinker sees alcohol as "pleasure-elixir." But Mr. Stop sees alcohol as "poison." Thus, in order to *get into more agreement*, and to *stop the inner war*, Mr. Drinker and Mr. Stop need to compromise, on a more "intermediate" definition of alcohol!

By regarding alcohol as "medicine," the compromise has been achieved, so that Mr. Drinker and Mr. Stop can finally cooperate! For "medicine" is about halfway between "pleasure-elixir" and "poison." Consider that many drugs, which doctors prescribe patients today as "medicine," are really closer to being "poisons." Also, carefully measuring out the amount of consumed "alcohol/medicine" and recording it in a notebook, is something that a scientist or doctor would do. The "alcohol/medicine" becomes more of a "prescription" by this process, similar to an actual medicine. But the

"Alcohol/medicine" still continues to affect the client pleasurably! Thus, a good compromise has been reached, between "pleasure-elixir" and "poison," in this intermediate term "medicine," or "alcohol/medicine"!

Once this clever method unites the warring parts of Mr. Drinker and Mr. Stop in a client, the gradual "weaning" progress can continue to where (day-by-day) less and less alcohol is consumed.

Either this method can be used to: 1) eventually quit alcohol altogether, or else 2) to *reduce* the daily measured-out "alcohol/medicine" down to a tolerable level that is no longer ruining the health and wrecking the life!

It's the *gratitude* of Mr. Drinker, that he's still allowed a little "alcohol/medicine" daily (as long as it's carefully measured out) that induces him (finally) to cooperate with Mr. Stop! Thus, together, *in unity*, they can *team up* to reduce the "alcohol/medicine" to a minimum, that no longer wrecks one's health and life!

Method #2 - The Hypnotic Extreme Disgust Method

This method involves your going into a hypnotic trance, and having numerous "true negatives" (about alcohol) suggested to you. The object is to fill you so full of "*ultra-disgust*" toward alcohol, that you'll stop drinking it.

With the hypnotic words of this method, possibility #1 is to record them into a recording device. Speaking slowly, in a monotone-like voice, helps greatly here. Then, later, when you're lying down, with eyes closed, and ready to be hypnotized, you can play all the recorded hypnotic words back, to yourself. Possibility #2 is to have *another person* (a friend) read—from this book—the hypnotic words to you when you're lying down with your eyes closed. Your friend should read the hypnotic words *slowly*! Either way is okay; it's up to you.

Before I write down the hypnotic words for you to use, it will greatly help for you to do a computer search for: "spittoon wild west saloon". Click on where it offers "spittoon *symbols*", then take a look at the pictures of actual, genuine *spittoons*, from the "wild west saloon" era. For, it will be *this spittoon* (in your imagination, while hypnotized) that you will disgustingly place your face in! This repulsive placing of your face into the spittoon (full of spit out alcohol, cowboy vomit, and mongrel dog urine) will be hypnotically associated with alcohol. And, this awful experience is designed to fill you full of *utter disgust toward alcohol* (to make you stop drinking it)!

So now, go ahead and just read these words, designed to (later!) hypnotize you. *See* whether you (later) want to put yourself through this "ultra-disgusting" hypnotic experience, in order to stop alcohol. (If you don't, that's okay. Simply go on to one of the other methods in this book.)

HYPNOTIC WORDS THAT YOU'LL BE (SLOWLY) RECORDING, OR THAT YOUR FRIEND WILL (SLOWLY) READ TO YOU:

"Relax your entire body. Your entire body feels completely comfortable and relaxed. Relax your *feet*. Your feet feel completely comfortable and relaxed. Relax your *legs*. Your legs feel completely comfortable, and relaxed. Relax your *hips*. Your hips feel completely comfortable and relaxed. Relax your *stomach*. Your stomach feels completely comfortable, and relaxed. Relax your *chest*. Your chest feels completely comfortable, and relaxed. Relax your *arms*. Your arms feel completely comfortable, and relaxed. Relax your *hands*. Relax your *fingers*. Relax your *neck & throat*. Your neck & throat feel completely comfortable, and relaxed. Relax your *face* and your *head*. Your face, and your head, feel completely comfortable, and relaxed. Relax your *eyes*. Relax your *mouth*. Relax your entire body. Your entire body feels completely comfortable and relaxed. And, every breath that you take, makes you feel more comfortable and relaxed. Just lie there, and feel how good it feels, to feel so comfortable and relaxed. And every breath that you take, makes you feel more and more comfortable, and more and more relaxed.

(Now, record all these 172 "relax-relax-relax" words all over again, a second time, before proceeding *onwards*.)

"*Now*, I want you to fully open your mind and emotions, all the way, in listening to all the *truths* I will now tell you about alcohol. I'm now going to tell you many, many *truths* about alcohol that will flow straight into your mind and emotions *without any resistance*. Okay, here I go. Now, *absorb fully* all I'm going to say *directly* to you, about alcohol, right now!"

Alcohol is really a *poison*! It's a toxic poison that destroys your health! Drinking alcohol, over time, gradually makes you more and more *sick*! Your liver, heart, digestive system, kidneys, brain, and many other body parts get gradually *destroyed*, by alcohol! So that your health, energy, and life get wrecked! Also, addiction turns you into an alcohol *slave*! Drinking alcohol leads to a heart attack, cancer, or death! Alcohol damages your whole body! Your whole life goes to hell, from drinking alcohol! The price tag, of drinking alcohol over a lifetime, is about $300,000! The way to be happy and feel good is to *not* drink alcohol! And you know all of this already! So, quit! Now that you see how horrible alcohol is, from all these reasons, you'll feel so *disgusted* from alcohol that you'll quit! Immediately! You'll completely stop alcohol right now! You'll feel so *disgusted* toward alcohol. Yes, you'll *stop*, and stop alcohol, right *now*!

(Now, record the last two paragraphs, of 225 words total, all over again, a second time, before proceeding further.)

"Okay, now I want you to imagine that you're back in the "wild west days", around the year 1880. And, imagine that you're in a wild west saloon, full of cowboys. Let your imagination take you back through time, to around the year 1880, where you're standing inside an old wild west saloon, full of cowboys."

(Pause 5 seconds.)

"Okay, now look towards the bar, of the saloon, and in the middle of the bar, on the floor, see an old wild west *spittoon*. See this dirty, old, stinking spittoon, on the floor, in the middle of the bar."

(Pause 5 seconds.)

"Now, notice how all the cowboys are frequently "hawking" and *spitting* into the spittoon, and are often spitting out jets of their yellowish spit, mixed with alcohol, into the spittoon. See that the spittoon's outer surface is all covered with disgusting spit, mixed with alcohol."

(Pause 5 seconds.)

"And notice also, that the drunken cowboys occasionally vomit up their alcohol, from over-drinking, into the spittoon. Because of that, the spittoon reeks with the stench of this cowboy vomit, mixed with alcohol."

(Pause 5 seconds.)

Finally, notice that there are a few filthy, ugly, mongrel dogs running around the saloon, and that these disgusting mongrel dogs occasionally lift their leg by the spittoon, and urinate their stinking dog piss, into the spittoon.

(Pause 5 seconds.)

"Now, I want you to ignore all the cowboys and mongrel dogs, and walk up to the spittoon, so that you're standing right in front of it, looking down at all of its filth."

(Pause 5 seconds.)

"And now, I want you to kneel down in front of the disgusting spittoon."

(Pause 5 seconds.)

"As you closely kneel, notice all the yellow spit, vomit, and dog piss, mixed with alcohol, swirling around disgustingly, in the stinking spittoon."

(Pause 5 seconds.)

"Now, all that you disgustingly see and smell, right in front of your face, you will *strongly associate* with drinking alcohol. *Do it! Do this association! Now!*"

(Pause 5 seconds.)

"So that, whenever in the future you're just about to drink alcohol, you'll also strongly experience all the disgust you now feel, from seeing and smelling all the disgusting yellow spit, vomit, alcohol, and dog piss, in this spittoon."

(Pause 5 seconds.)

"And now, push your face into the awful spit, vomit, alcohol, and dog piss, as you *fully experience* the *awfulness* of *drinking alcohol!*"

(Pause 5 seconds.)

"Feel some of the spit, vomit, alcohol, and dog piss get in your nose and mouth, as you strongly associate all this with drinking alcohol!"

(Pause 5 seconds.)

"Okay, enough! *The experience is over*! You're here in the present, again. The cowboy saloon of 1880 is back in the past, and you're here again, in the present. Your face is *no longer* in the spittoon, and your face, nose, and mouth no longer have any spit or vomit or alcohol, or dog piss in, or on, them; they're *clean!*"

(Pause 5 seconds.)

"But your memory of this disgust will remain strong! You will *strongly associate drinking alcohol* with all the disgust of the memory of your face in the spittoon."

(Pause 5 seconds.)

"So that, every time you want to drink alcohol, the disgusting memory of your face in the spittoon will be *so strong* that it will *completely stop you from drinking alcohol!*"

(Pause 5 seconds.)

"Because you will *strongly* associate drinking alcohol with the disgusting memory of your face in the spittoon, you'll never drink alcohol again!"

(Pause 5 seconds.)

"In fact, right now, you feel such tremendous disgust towards drinking alcohol, that *right now, you absolutely know that you will never drink alcohol again*! Feel, right now, this *ultra-disgust of drinking alcohol*, so strong in you, that you know you will never drink alcohol again! Feel it! *Strongly! Now!*"

(Pause 5 seconds.)

"After I bring you out of this hypnotic trance, you will *clearly remember* all the *extreme negatives* of drinking alcohol that flowed straight into your mind and emotions without any resistance. You will especially remember that drinking alcohol is so especially toxic and poisonous, that you *must* stop drinking alcohol!"

(Pause 5 seconds.)

"Also, whenever any time in the future, you're about to take *any action* toward resuming drinking alcohol, you'll strongly experience the disgusting memory of your face in the sickening spittoon, of spit, vomit, alcohol, and dog piss. This returning memory will be so ultra-disgusting, that no drinking of alcohol will happen, and *you'll never, ever, drink alcohol again*! I repeat, you will *never, ever, drink alcohol again!*"

(Pause 5 seconds.)

"I'm now about to wake you up, from this hypnotic trance. And, after I do you'll feel fine, rested, and refreshed. I'm going to count back from 5 to 1. And as I count back, you'll slowly wake up. So, "5", you're starting to wake up. And, "4", you're waking up even more. And, "3", you're halfway awake. And, "2", you're almost awake, feeling fine, rested, and refreshed. And, "1!" (*clapping of hands, loudly, here*). You're *awake*, feeling fine, rested and refreshed!

(THIS IS THE END OF THE HYPNOTIC SPEECH.)

Note #1. About 95% of the time, the hypnotic subject *will* wake up from the hypnosis, after you say: "1!", and clap your hands loudly. But, about 5% of the time, they won't wake up. If they don't wake up, then shake them gently, and say their name loudly, followed by "Wake up!" This should do it. But if they still won't wake up, then just leave them be. They'll just fall into a normal sleep or nap, and eventually wake up later, on their own. There is nothing to worry about if this happens! Alternatively, you could wait *ten minutes, then shake them again, calling out their name.*

Note #2. Because the hypnotic speech is either in your *own* voice (on a recording device), or read to you in your *friend's* voice, it probably will be *very powerful.* Possibly, even more powerful than a professional hypnotist's voice, because you intuitively *trust* your own voice and your friend's voice! Also, it's even possible to repeatedly hypnotize yourself (with this hypnotic speech) *every day* (if you want to). Obviously, frequent repetition, of this hypnotic speech, makes it stronger. I suppose it might be okay to change or alter some of the wording, but only if you know what you're doing (because you, yourself, are a semi-professional). Be extremely careful here! All of this hypnotic *wording is going straight into your subconscious mind*!

Note #3. You can delete all words referring to the mongrel dogs and their piss, if this too utterly grosses you out. But if your drinking doesn't stop, add it back it, perhaps!

Method #3 - Self-Hypnosis To Take You To An "Inner Guide" Or "Wise Part Of Yourself" Instead

It's also possible to use the 172 "relax-relax-relax" words (from Method #2, the first paragraph of HYPNOTIC WORDS) *only* (repeated twice). After this, record suggestions that you'll go (inwardly) to an "inner guide" (or wise part of yourself), who will then tell you how *you* can best stop drinking alcohol! This method (or perhaps a combination of methods) may be the *most effective* for you!

In this revised hypnotic speech, after you've had about *five minutes of silence* (to receive your wise messages inwardly), then record (on this revised hypnotic recording) the "waking up" words of counting from "5" to "1".

You can try this *alternative* self-hypnosis instead!

Method #4 - The Banishing Alcohol Method

With common "twelve-step programs", you usually call on a Higher Power, to help you to stop. This Banishing Alcohol Method uses a similar strategy, in calling on the same Higher Power, but in a different, more-direct, and personal way.

There exists a very ancient system of higher knowledge and wisdom called the *Cabala*. Of the Cabala's many teachings and rituals, a very, very powerful "rubric ritual" is called the "Lesser Banishing Ritual of the Pentagram". This rubric ritual is *absolutely ideal* for banishing something bad from your life, like drinking alcohol.

Now, in doing rituals, you do *not* need a lot of expensive equipment and paraphernalia in order to make the ritual work! Rituals work because of the *"Power of Intention"* of the worker of the ritual. So, my instructions for doing the rubric ritual (to banish alcohol from your life) will only involve *inexpensive* props. If you want to add more elaborate or expensive props, you can try:

1. a special, meaningful robe,

2. some kind of altar,

3. a candle,

4. a more-elaborate or expensive wand,

5. a symbolized pentagram or special rug,

6. an elaborate headpiece,

7. meaningful jewelry,

8. ritual dance (for example, a special "Stop Alcohol Dance" you create),

9. posters or symbols on the walls (perhaps something you create),

10. a room specially set aside only for rituals,

11. appropriate music (perhaps your own recorded "Stop Alcohol Song" or "Stop Alcohol Chant" that you've created),

12. aroma-therapies or flower essences that increase your "Power of Intention",

13. crystals,

14. Tibetan singing bowls,

15. drumming, flute playing, or playing any instrument you choose,

16. lunar timing (starting at the new moon, etc.),

17. ritual nudity,

18. an ashtray stuffed with smoked butts (symbolizing quitting?) resting on a crushed cigarette pack, perhaps,

19. anything else you can think of, to increase the power of this "Banishing-alcohol Ritual".

Incidentally, rituals are *"advanced working psychology"*, and are somewhat similar to self-hypnosis. In rituals, you are sort of "putting a spell" on yourself or your subconscious mind (in this case, to stop alcohol). "Part A" (the part of you that wants to quit) is "putting a ritualistic spell" on "Part B" (the part of you that *won't* quit)! Every day we go through this dichotomy naturally, where different parts of our personality struggle to get their way (over other, opposite, parts of our personality). So, this is all just basic-basic psychology, really. Doing a ritual is just taking it one step further. It's simply more *powerful* to use self-hypnosis, affirmations, chanting, meditating, aromatherapies, yoga, t'ai chi, trance-dance, counseling, religion, 12-step programs, or *rituals*, to stop an out-of-control part of our personality from *wrecking our life by alcohol*!

For this ritual, you could use a wand or ritual dagger. Or, you could just use your extended fore-finger, instead.

Instructions for Rubric Ritual

1. Face *East*, in the middle of a room, or in front of your altar (optional).

2. Have your wand nearby for later, and ready to pick it up quickly.

3. Touch your forehead, and say (aloud): *"ATAH!"* (Hebrew for "Thou Art").

4. Touch your solar plexus, and say (aloud): *"MALKUTH!"* (Hebrew for "The Kingdom").

5. Touch your *right* shoulder and say (aloud):*"VE-GEVURAH!"* (Hebrew for "And the Power").

6. Touch your *left* shoulder and say (aloud):*"VE-GEDULAH!"* (Hebrew for "And the Glory").

7. Join your palms together in the common "praying" gesture (fingers pointing up). Put your joined palms over the exact middle of your chest (heart chakra), and say (aloud): *"LE-OLAHM, AMEN!"* (Hebrew for "Forever, Amen").

7. Pick up your wand (from nearby) and hold it in your dominant hand.

8. Draw a huge five-armed star (a *pentagram*) in the air, with your wand. Imagine the star flaming blue fire, as you draw it. Start at the lower left (1), then move your wand diagonally upward (about four feet) to the star's top-most point (2). Then, move your wand diagonally down to the star's lower right point (3). Then move your wand to the star's left-side point (4). Then, to the star's right-side point (5). Finally, move your wand back diagonally down to the starting point, at the lower left (1). The star is now drawn! All the while, as you draw it, imagine it flaming, in blue fire, in the air! (See next page for a drawing.)

9. Stab the star in its middle with your wand, and say (assertively): *"YOD-HEH-VAV-HEH!"* (This,

incidentally, is one of the most powerfully manifesting ritualistic words that exists, as this is the highest Hebrew expression for God's name.)

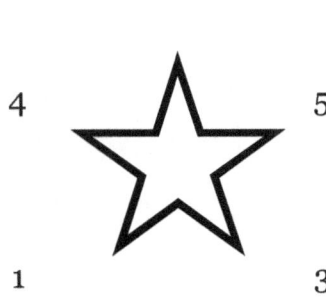

10. Turn clockwise (to your right), and face *South*. Draw a second star (of flaming blue fire) in the air, as before, stab it in the center, and say (assertively): "*AH-DOH-NAI!*" (Another Hebrew expression, meaning "My Lord", used only for God.)

11. Turn clockwise and face *West*. Draw a third star (of flaming blue fire) in the air, as before, stab it in the center, and say (assertively): "*EH-YEH!*" (Yet another Hebrew name for God.)

12. Turn clockwise, and face *North*. Draw a fourth star (of flaming blue fire) in the air, as before, stab it in the center, and say (assertively): "*AH-GAH-LAH!*"(A Hebrew acronym for "*ATAH GIBOR LE-OLAHM ADONAI*", meaning "You, O Lord, are mighty forever", used as a name of God.)

13. Turn clockwise (to complete the circle) and Face *East* again (as you started).

14. Hold your arms straight out to the sides, with your wand still in your hand (so that your body forms a cross), and say:

   "BEFORE ME IS RAPHAEL

   "BEHIND ME IS GABRIEL

   "TO MY RIGHT IS MICHAEL

   "AND TO MY LEFT IS ARIEL

   "ABOUT ME FLAME THE PENTAGRAMS

   "AND ABOVE ME SHINES THE POWER AND GLORY OF GOD!"

16. Then say:

   "ARCHANGEL RAPHAEL! ARCHANGEL GABRIEL!

   "ARCHANGEL MICHAEL! ARCHANGEL ARIEL!

   "GOD, WITH ALL YOUR POWER AND GLORY!

   "PLEASE, HELP ME TO STOP ALCOHOL, AS QUICKLY AS POSSIBLE!

   "PLEASE, I AM ASKING FOR YOUR HELP!"

17. Intensely *feel* as much *desire* as you possibly can, that you will stop drinking alcohol!

18. Then, intensely *feel* as much *triumph* as you possibly can, as you feel strongly confident that you actually will stop!

19. And then, stand there, for about a minute, and *feel* the incredible *spiritual power* of the four highest archangels, and God, empowering you to stop drinking alcohol. (If your arms get tired, you can bend them a

little, to ease the strain of holding them straight out. You can cup your palms a bit, to receive the Highest Energy from the four archangels and God.)

20. Put down your wand, at the nearby spot where you had it at the start.

21. Touch your forehead, and say (aloud): "*ATAH!*"

22. Touch your solar plexus, and say (aloud): "*MALKUTH!*"

23. Touch your *right* shoulder and say (aloud):"*VE-GEVURAH!*"

24. Touch your *left* shoulder and say (aloud):"*VE-GEDULAH!*"

25. Join your palms together in the common "praying" gesture (fingers pointing up). Put your joined palms over the exact middle of your chest (heart chakra), and say (aloud): "*LE-OLAHM, AMEN!*" (This completes the rubric ritual.)

Aftermath. Feel the powerful effects of this rubric ritual awhile, either as you just stand there, or go and sit down, or lie down. You may feel very spiritual, from your contact with the four archangels and God. You may feel other feelings, or sensations, and it would be good to write all this down in a special notebook, or "Ritual Diary". Also, write down any insights that may come to you, that may creatively help you to stop drinking alcohol. These insights and intuitions *could* be very important spiritual messages coming from the four archangels and God, to facilitate your stopping alcohol! Be sure to write them down!

Note. If you live in a thin-walled place, where neighbors can easily hear you, it's okay to whisper or softly mumble all the ritual's words. The powerfulness of your *intention* is what's important, not necessarily the loudness of your words!

Doing this rubric ritual daily should greatly help you to quit drinking alcohol! You are asking the *Highest Spiritual Forces In The Universe* to help you to quit drinking alcohol! Thus, this method is similar to a twelve-step program. The difference is that you can contact God and the four archangels yourself, directly, whenever you want, so that you're creating a personal, intimate relationship with God and the four archangels, as they help you to stop drinking alcohol.

Because this "little" rubric ritual seems so "simple" and "brief", many, many people have *completely underestimated its power*! Actually, it's one of the most powerful working rituals ever devised by mankind! For, what could be more powerful than contacting God and the four chief archangels, using all the super-powerful words that are spoken in this rubric ritual?

This Banishing Method can be combined with any other methods to stop drinking alcohol. But, *especially* combine it with any intuitions, insights, ideas, or guidance received from God at the conclusion of the rubric ritual. (Write all this down, in your "Ritual Diary").

Go ahead and *try* this rubric ritual, and you'll be *amazed* to find out how incredibly well it *works*!

[**Caution.** If this ritual doesn't seem to be working after 10 tries, then discontinue it! Afterward, if "God" or any "Archangels" seem to start talking *back* to you, ignore them or tell them to stop. This is because most likely they're autonomous psychological entities you may have created with this ritual. Obviously, *you* need to decide how to live your life, not voices from the subconscious calling themselves "God" or by a name of one the Archangels. Also, anyone with a history of mental illness may need to avoid this method.]

Method #5 - Quit in 3 Months, on Birthday

Sam decided, three months before turning 50, that it would be a good time to quit, at age 50. Also, because his birthday was on January 1st, in line with new year's resolutions, it really felt like the perfect time to do it, for him.

Sam was sick and tired of feeling rotten every morning when he woke up, because he had gone to bed drunk. Each "hungover" morning, he forgot almost all that had happened the previous day. Sam forgot who he had talked to, what he had said, and what had happened with others, etc. He was always worried that he had said or done the wrong thing, yesterday, and then forgotten all this, due to drunkenness.

"Did I make a total ass of myself?" Sam would wonder. "Was my being drunk embarrassing in any way?" he'd question. "What in the heck really *did* happen yesterday?" Sam pondered.

So, Sam decided, three months before turning 50 (on New Year's Day), that he would quit on January 1st. First, he told all his friends and acquaintances that he was stopping all alcohol drinking on January 1st. Then people would know there was to be no more drinking on his part, and wouldn't be expecting Sam to drink with them, any more. Also, if Sam didn't follow through with quitting on January 1st, then everyone would think that Sam was a liar, or weak. This would greatly humiliate and embarrass Sam.

Second, Sam realized, in the last 3 months before quitting, that since he wouldn't be drinking any more after January 1st, he'd better take *full advantage* of alcohol, and get drunk every night, even more than usual! So, Sam got (in his own words) "shit-faced drunk" every night, for the next 3 months!

Sam actually forced himself to drink and drink, and drink, until he passed out. "One more," "one more," he kept saying to himself. But then, Sam found that by forcing all that beer on himself, he got sick of drinking beer. In fact, by continually forcing an overdose of beer on himself every night, Sam got so sick of beer that he began to very much *want* to drink no more!

Finally, on January 1st, Sam's 50th birthday, Sam woke up feeling great. And, it felt totally right to stop alcohol drinking at this point. It felt so good to no longer be making an ass of himself, drunk. No longer would Sam be spending $12 a day on beer. This would save $4,000 per year (365 x $12). Sam could spend it instead on "all kinds of neat stuff," he thought, enthusiastically.

Sam discovered that he had so much extra energy in the morning now, after quitting beer! He put all this enormous new energy into doing lots and lots of things he liked. As an analogy, Sam realized that the way to stop chocolate cake addiction was to eat chocolate cake until you "puked." Then, sickened by this, one doesn't want sugar or chocolate cake, any more!

Sam totally realized that looking stupid to people (when drunk) was *not fun*, at all. Sam realized that, when drunkenly slurring words, he looked like an idiot.

Now that Sam had completely stopped drinking, he realized that he shouldn't tell people he'll "not drink forever," because whenever one says that, the contrary rebellious urge comes up, to do the opposite, and to do what you say you'll *not* do. So instead, Sam tells people, "I'm stopping *for now*!"

Also, whenever Sam finds himself craving beer, he says to himself, "I don't want a beer." As he says this, he does it with the *full realization* of all the negatives that come with the beer drinking that he *doesn't want*. Thus, when Sam says to himself, "I don't want a beer," *it's true*, because he *really doesn't* want a beer because of its *inseparable connection* with all of the *negatives* that come with it!

Sam is now 53, and he has been completely alcohol-free for 3 years.

So, the gist of this method is: 1) Pick a *quit date*; 2) Three months before this quit date, do what Sam did; or, 3) Alter this method in any way that tailors it to your own unique personality, and what works for you! Re-design it all, to work for you, then quit!

Method #6 - 6-A-Day Limit

My friend Tony was in his fifties, and had been drinking alcohol for thirty years. He knew that dire health problems could begin, if he didn't quit, at his age.

Tony still enjoyed drinking a certain amount, however. So Tony decided on a plan to limit himself to *six* beers a day. But every day, after his sixth beer, Tony continued to drink several more, and averaged about fifteen beers a day (instead of six). However, this still was better than the twenty beers Tony used to drink, every day!

After Tony's sixth beer, he usually tried as hard as he could, with all his willpower, to stop for the day. So that, even though Tony drank several more beers than six, he was still "exercising" his willpower "muscles," by trying to stop at six!

Half a year passed like this, and Tony became very disappointed in himself for "failing" every day, to stop at six beers only. At this point, Tony decided that his "6-A-Day Limit" system just wasn't working. But he still knew that he needed to quit for health reasons.

Tony, at this point, decided to go "cold turkey." Not knowing of any other systems to stop alcohol, Tony made a "capital D" *D*ecision to totally stop. And, he did! He was able, at this point, to completely stop drinking, and he had very few alcohol withdrawal problems, and is still not drinking alcohol today, after all these years. So, Tony did it. He stopped!

Perhaps Tony's exercising of his willpower "muscles," every day for six months, developed these "muscles" enough so that Tony's willpower (after six months of growing stronger) was finally strong enough for him to quit drinking alcohol altogether!

Note. This method can be used with a lesser number of beers per day, or with glasses of wine per day, or even with hard liquor drinks per day. Just follow the same strategy (or a very similar strategy) as Tony did with beer.

Method #7 - Quit or Die

My friend Andy's favorite hobby was going to the local drag strip, to watch the cars race and help out in the pit. All his friends were there drinking lots of beer, laughing, joking, and partying. What great fun it all was!

Then, after a physical exam at age 49, Andy was diagnosed by his doctor as having early signs of stomach cancer. Andy's doctor told him—in no uncertain terms—that Andy *must* stop his drinking, or die! Understandably, this greatly shocked Andy and forced him to do some very deep thinking.

Now, Andy *loved* watching drag racing. And he *loved* drinking beer with his buddies. What to do? It would be just too awkward to go to the drag strip and *not* drink beer, while all his friends were chugging it down.

Andy finally decided to *experiment* with drinking "near beer" at the drag strip. That way, he could still have the "taste" of alcohol, as he drank along with his buddies. (Naturally, Andy informed his friends why he needed to drink the "near beer," instead.)

Andy went through his doctor's treatment for stomach cancer and survived. He fully understood that alcohol could easily cause a relapse of the cancer. Thus, Andy still sticks to "near beer," while passionately enjoying his hobby and friends, at the drag strip. (An alternative that you might consider would be non-alcoholic wine.)

Here is the *essence* of this method:

You don't need to wait for your doctor to give you a "health ultimatum." You know that alcohol is slowly killing you, and it's only a *matter of time* before you're gravely threatened by some deadly disease. So, why wait as long as Andy? Why risk some disease or operation, etc., killing you? You know when you are a heavy drinker, it's probably *absolutely inevitable*. Incidentally, walking in *graveyards* can really help here to *force* you to face that alcohol *truly* is killing you!

What to do:

(1) Make a simple drawing of your favorite alcohol beverage. Then draw an arrow from it, pointing to the right. Then, draw your own dead corpse! When all this is drawn (however crudely) by yourself, it will be *much more powerful* than someone else's (perhaps more professional) drawing.

(2) Hold your drawing in front of your eyes, very close to your face.

(3) As you stare at your drawing, *get* that *this is reality.* Alcohol is a poison and most likely, in the long run, it will kill you! (Perhaps bringing your drawing to a graveyard, to view it as you walk the graveyard, will double its power.)

(4) Feel the fear, shock, and horror, as the reality *sinks in,* that toxic alcohol will kill you. Really! No joke, here!

(5) Change, as Andy chose to, from drinking alcohol to some alternative. Perhaps near beer or non-alcoholic wine, or one of dozens of alternatives listed in other methods of this book.

(6) Any time you crave alcohol, put your drawing in front of your face again; feel the fear, shock, and horror again, then either skip the drink, or drink only *half* as much alcohol (your choice).

(7) By this method, *realistic* fear (of alcohol killing you) should *at least* reduce alcohol to only 50%, which is very significant!

Method #8 - The Furious Anger Method

(By Ted, who drank alcohol for 20 years.)

Ted stopped alcohol (finally) with anger! He got *really angry* about all the negatives of alcohol. Angry about the expense of alcohol. Angry about being an alcohol addict. Angry about the alcohol stinking up his breath. Angry about it wrecking his health. Angry that alcohol could eventually kill him. Angry about his constantly craving a drink so much. But especially, angry towards all the people who wanted him to quit!

Ted took his *utter volcano of anger*, and turned it towards alcohol itself! Ted was so angry about all the negatives of alcohol, and so *absolutely fed up*, with all the negatives of alcohol, that he turned his furious, raging anger towards alcohol itself, and was thus able to quit!

For, when furious, boiling anger, that fills your whole being, becomes so incredibly big that you want to kill or destroy something, then it's a very, very powerful thing. And, if you can then turn that powerful, voluminous anger towards something *bad*, then you can destroy that bad thing! And, that's what Ted did. He took his ultra-enormous anger, and directed it towards alcohol itself, and thus was able to quit!

Note. Furious boiling anger can be worked up easier by: 1) putting on a pair of *red* color therapy glasses, or 2) putting on a pair of "brain hemisphere glasses" (described in Method #33, Love Yourself Method) that are the *opposite* of what is recommended in Method #33, so that you'll be stimulating your *angriest* brain hemisphere! Then, put the red color therapy glasses *over* the brain hemisphere glasses, to catapult yourself into what the British describe as a "very fine rage"!

Also, 3) make use of *any* technique you can think of, to *drive* yourself into an "ultra-intense rage." Perhaps play punk rock music that you *especially hate*? Or, smell your least-favorite smells? Maybe repeatedly snap a rubber band that you have put around your wrist? Anyway, work up a tremendous ultra-rage, then redirect this rage towards alcohol itself, to then stop it!

Method #9 - Affirm Quit Date Repeatedly As One Drinks Alcohol Heavily And Excessively

A friend of mine, Paul, successfully quit in the following way. For a whole year, from Jan. 1 to Dec. 31, he drank alcohol heavily and even *excessively*. But, as he gulped down each alcohol drink, he affirmed, with certainty "I will be quitting on January 1st" (of the next year).

Thus, hundreds of times a day for 365 straight days, *with each alcohol beverage he drank*, he fervently declared, over and over, his *conviction* to quit at the beginning of the next year. Finally, when January 1st of the next year came, all his passionate affirming paid off, and he quit!

Affirmations like this can be *greatly empowered* by (1) rapidly moving your eyes from side to side, as described in Beaulieu's book "Eye Movement Integration Therapy," or (2) making and using "Glasses A" and "Glasses B" as described in Method #33 (Love Yourself Method).

Method #10 - Dream Solution

Before going to bed at night, write down these words, and put them under your pillow: "I wish for my dream tonight to inspire me with the *best solution*, for me to stop alcohol!" (Word this message in your own way, if you want.)

After you put your "dream solution message" under your pillow, feel *extreme desire* for this to happen. You can light a candle, look at the candle, and *feel burning desire* that you'll receive (in your dream) guidance, of what's the best way for you to stop alcohol! (A white or light blue candle might work best.)

Then, feel *extreme triumph*, the "winning feeling", as if *you have already received* (from the dream) the guidance of how to best stop alcohol! Then, put out the candle, and retire for the night.

If you wake up in the middle of the night (or in the morning) with your dream's "stop alcohol solution", be sure to write it down! (Have pen and paper, and a light, easily reachable from your bed.) Or, if after a week of trying this every night, you still haven't received a "guidance dream", then try taking some *herbs* that stimulate dreaming, before going to sleep. Do an Internet search on "dreaming herbs that stimulate dreaming", to find herbs that seem to be best for this, or try the "Dream Enhancer" formula of 1/8 teaspoon each of the dried herbs: valerian, hops, and skullcap. Or, you can buy a Native American "dreamcatcher" talisman, which also could help; search online for this, too! Finally, if you just can't seem to induce a guiding dream in these ways, then use this method to induce a guiding daydream. Just let your mind spontaneously daydream, then record the daydreams in a notebook, for later interpretation.

Method #11 - Lucid Dreaming

The Lucid Dreaming method is based on the possibility that your own *personal* answer, of how to best stop alcohol, may simply *lie within* you!

Lucid dreaming is where, in a dream that you are having, you "wake up in the dream." When this happens, you are as *awake* and *conscious* in the "dream world" as you normally are in this regular, everyday, physical world. It's quite a surprise and adventure, this "waking up in your dream world." Unfortunately, it usually only lasts a few seconds, before you find yourself *actually* waking up, in bed. You see, the *shock* of waking up in your dream often speedily results in an *actual* waking up, in bed (unfortunately).

This method involves (a) waking up in your dream, (b) resisting (successfully) an actual waking up in bed, then (c) searching in this "lucid-dream world" for a guru, wise person, shaman, book of wisdom, symbol, or *anything else*, that will tell you (or indicate allegorically to you) how *you* (personally) can best stop alcohol!

There are several books on lucid dreaming available, in libraries or on the internet, that you can get to learn and practice the methods involved. My favorite method, one I've successfully practiced many times, is in Ophiel's book, *The Art and Practice of Astral Projection*. In this book, Ophiel's "dream method" leads to waking up in your dream (after a bit of practicing the book's techniques).

(1) First, you go around in the regular, everyday, physical world looking for anything *extremely weird*, like a person with two heads, a flying cat, or blood-colored rain, etc. Obviously, you won't see any of this, but you *get in the habit* of fervently searching for weirdness, with the intention of *concluding you are dreaming* if you see it!

(2) This habit will then "carry over" into your dreams, so that in your dreams, you'll also find yourself "fervently looking for weirdness." Except, in your dreams, you'll really *find* this weirdness, and when you do, and then quickly conclude that you're dreaming, then *yes*, you really are dreaming! At this point, you'll actually wake up in your dream!

(3) But often here, within seconds, you'll just wake up in bed, unless you are also fervently pre-practicing this next step:

(4) Whenever you wake up in bed from a dream, strongly will yourself to "return to the dream" as fervently as you can. That is, sort of dream it over again, as vividly as possible. You almost certainly *won't* actually get back to the dream state this way, but you'll be *developing and strengthening the* "return muscles" *in your* brain! As these "return muscles" become stronger and *stronger*, you're then ready for the situation at the end of step (2), above: When you actually "wake up in your dream," you'll then use your greatly strengthened "return muscles" to *return to the dream*, but since *you're actually still in your dream*, you'll . . .

(5) *Stay there*, instead of waking up in bed! Then . . .

(6) Awake in your dream (and staying there, in your dream), you search for your personal "Stop Alcohol Solution."

Get Ophiel's book (or another lucid dreaming book) and try all this! (You might need to re-read these instructions a few more times, to thoroughly understand all this.)

Lucid Daydreaming can also work, too. In a daydreamy state, gently direct the daydreamy inner world towards finding a wise entity who can give to you, your own personal "stop alcohol" solution! Jung calls this technique "Active Imagination." In Eckankar (started by Paul Twitchell) this technigue is expertly taught. Search for Jung's "Active Imagination", or "Eckankar" on the internet. (Jung repeatedly states that imagination is the source of all creative solutions.)

Method #12 - Aerobic Shape

Several friends of mine, who used to have trouble with depression, told me that once they got in *aerobic shape*, they "waved their blues goodbye." This is because emotions are *very connected* with our endocrine system and bodily organs, etc. Just look at children and all the other mammals. Notice how *emotional* they are, and how their emotions are very connected to the movements and activities of their body, as they rapidly and actively move about!

Since depression is a fairly big factor in why people drink alcohol, then *stopping depression with aerobic shape* can really help to stop *alcohol.* You'll be removing a *big* part of the cause! By eliminating or greatly reducing depression (with aerobic shape), you'll stand an excellent chance of eliminating or greatly reducing alcohol, too!

But you *must* exercise with an activity that you *really like*! This is ultra-important! Otherwise, the odds are that you *just won't stick with it.* Why should you, if a type of activity *bores* you, or you just *don't like it*?

Compile a list of 100 different ways to exercise, using the internet. You'll be *amazed* at how many ways there are to get in aerobic shape! Then, put a (1), (2), and (3) by your top three choices. These (1), (2), and (3) should be the ways that are the *most fun* for you! So, these activities will then be what works for you!

Of course, if it turns out that *none* of these 100 ways of exercising appeal to you, then joining a gym may be necessary. Then, when you arrive at the gym and see everyone else exercising, you'll be motivated by simple "crowd psychology" to join in!

Anyway, give "aerobic shape exercising" a chance, to stop or cut down any *depression*, which will greatly help to cut down or stop *alcohol*!

Method #13 - Strongest Muscles Press

There is a system called "Bodynamics," invented by Peter Bernhardt in Oakland and Berkeley, California, around 1980. (There may still be some books out on it.)

The essence of this system is that all the muscles in your entire body's Muscular System can be organized into seven groups as:

(Category 1) Very Strong

(Category 2) Strong

(Category 3) Above Average in Strength

(Category 4) Average Strength

(Category 5) Below Average in Strength

(Category 6) Weak

(Category 7) Very Weak

Bodynamics was intended to go beyond Wilhelm Reich's system of healing so-called muscular armoring, in order to even more-effectively heal any chronic tension in the muscles.

However, this author has found by experience, that when massaging and pressing Category 1 - Very Strong muscles, then great willpower and personality strength is *temporarily* produced. *This great willpower can be tapped to stop the urge to drink alcohol, when it arises*!

This author's strongest muscles turned out to be the arm's biceps, along with the trapezius muscles (they're along the top of the shoulders, from the neck to the shoulder blades, and are used to "shrug the shoulders"). Whenever a noxious chore arose, this author would vigorously massage both biceps and both trapezius muscles. The resultant "great strength of will" that resulted (for about 30 seconds) would be used to plunge into the odious chore and "do it anyway."

This author personally discovered his very strongest muscles by systematically pressing almost every muscle and recording its "strength category" on a Bodynamics Chart (of 1980). Any reader interested in finding his very strongest muscles (to massage or press for bursts of super willpower) can try this same investigative *charting technique*. Go ahead and make up your own body-and-muscles chart, to record all your strengths, on your own, if you like.

Incidentally, I did tons of chin-ups on a backyard chin-up bar, as a kid, to develop super-strong biceps. And I later, in adolescence and in my 20s and 30s, did enormous weight-lifting to develop strong trapezius muscles, pectorals (chest), and front deltoids (between biceps and top of shoulder). I sometimes massage or press the pectorals or front deltoids, too, for great bursts of will and personality strength. Also, the acupuncture "Three More Miles" point can be pressed. It's below the knee, but on the outside of the shin bone. Press in, from the outside, against the shin bone, below both knees, for extra energy when you need it. *Thus, a shortcut to finding your strongest muscles can be massaging the muscles you've made strongest in sports or weight-lifting, and seeing how it makes you feel when these muscles are massaged!*

So, this is how it could work: Whenever alcohol craving strikes, quickly massage or press your strongest muscles, to give you (temporarily) Super Will, to resist the alcohol urge. Then quickly do something else (besides the alcohol) as a distraction. Have this *strategy* all worked out in advance, so that when alcohol craving strikes, you can quickly deflect it!

Method #14 - St. John's Wort

These are all the ways that St. John's Wort can help:

1) It soothes alcohol withdrawal symptoms.

2) It helps quench alcohol cravings.

3) It calms and relaxes.

4) It increases dopamine levels, to offset cravings. (Dopamine is a body chemical that induces happy moods.)

5) It helps eliminate toxins in your blood that were introduced there by alcohol.

6) It restores the balance between serotonin and dopamine in the brain.

7) It has hypericin, which is its most-significant ingredient. It's hypericin that's one of the main causative factors in reducing alcohol cravings.

8) It treats anxiety, melancholy, and depression.

9) It helps insomnia and nervousness.

10) Since depression often is one of the main causes of drinking alcohol, and since St. John's Wort very

effectively treats depression, then St. John's Wort will also tend to reduce or stop the drinking of alcohol.

Method #15 - Switch to Marijuana

I realize that some readers may be shocked at the above title, but really there are many big advantages to *smoking pot* instead of drinking booze. And remember: you *don't* have to switch 100%! You can still do *half* booze and half pot. Or one-quarter booze and three-quarters pot. Or even 1/8 booze and 7/8 pot! Some people even like booze and pot *together*. But watch out: you *don't* want to switch to 100% booze and *another* 100% pot! This method should only be done if the health-harming booze *really is reduced* and replaced by pot. Definitely don't do it, if you still do 100% booze, then add pot to this.

First, the disadvantages of this:

Problem (1) Pot is illegal, most places. *Solutions*: (a) Move to a state where it's legal, or where at least you can get "medical marijuana," somehow. (b) Don't move, but learn how and where to buy it safely and not get caught. Usually, if you buy *less than an ounce*, penalties are negligible (if caught). (c) Consider learning how to grow just a little of it (outdoors or indoors). Perhaps, in your state, you could get a medical marijuana permit, then grow *only* as many plants as allowed. (d) Befriend a pot seller or grower, then ask him lots of questions about all of this, to get *realistic* answers for *your area*!

Problem (2) Pot doesn't work as well as booze in getting you high. *Solutions*: (a) Smoke *more* pot, to "get you there." (b) Do some research on "pot enhancers"—ways to increase your high—from pot. Ask your "pot buddies" about this! (c)

Even if you reduce your booze to 75% (with 25% pot), it will still be better for your health than with 100% booze.

Problem (3) Pot makes you paranoid, gives you nausea or headaches, or has other negative effects (along with the high). *Solution*: Do some research on how to stop (or cut way down) on the paranoia, nausea, headaches, or other bad side effect of pot. Do an internet search on "stop paranoia," "stop nausea," "stop headaches," etc. Look for herbal remedies, or any other techniques, for this. Ask pot sellers or growers about this; do *they* know, from all their experience, of any ways to stop pot-induced paranoia, nausea, headaches, or whatever other bad pot-induced-side-effect you're experiencing? If you persist in your search-for-answers here, you should find some remedies eventually. Consider striking up conversations (about all this) with *many* pot sellers or growers. Remember, they'll be *very motivated* to give you some answers here! They'll very much *want you* to successfully switch from booze to pot, so that you'll become *their* regular client!

Problem (4) Your job requires regular urine tests for pot. *Solution*: There are "kits" you can buy for this. Ask around, especially pot sellers or growers.

The Advantages of Switching from Booze to Pot

(1) No more hangovers!

(2) No more danger in driving.

(3) No more risk of D.U.I.'s, etc.

(4) You'll no longer be wrecking your liver, heart, digestive system, or other organs and be headed for *death*!

(5) You'll stop destroying your brain and heading for *dementia*!

(6) No more *drunkenness* (along with all the problems connected with this).

(7) Your health will improve, noticeably.

(8) You'll have more self-respect.

(9) Many other (more subtle) benefits will result that you didn't expect!

So, what do you *think and feel*, from reading all this? Do you want to try switching from booze to pot? I hope that you don't think it'll turn you into a "hippie" or "commie" or anything like that. No! You're simply switching from one "recreational drug" (booze) to another (pot). That's all! You'll still be the same person, but just using *pot* instead of *booze*. And finding the successfully working ways to *make this switch happen*, to your liking!

Almost all the other methods in this book involve the *stopping* of booze. This method is *unique* in that here it's more of a *stop-and-start*, simultaneously. You'll *stop* booze, but you'll also *start* pot. And it can be done *gradually*, too:

Week 1: 75% booze and 25% pot.

Week 2: 50% booze and 50% pot.

Week 3: 25% booze and 75% pot.

Week 4: 0% booze (!) and 100% pot.

Note: It's possible to go *even slower* than this, with 90%, 80%, 70%, 60%, 50%, 40%, 30%, 20%, 10%, 0%!

Don't worry, you *won't* become any kind of hippie or commie (or anything else negative) from this switching from booze to pot (either 100% or just partway). Instead, you'll be a *hero*, who saved your own health and life!

Method #16 - Mixing Lots of Fruity Drinks

Once a friend of mine was offered a provocative-tasting drink that (supposedly) was alcoholic. He proceeded to drink and drink it, until he was quite "high." Then he was told that, really, the drink *wasn't* alcoholic, at all! He had been getting "high" on his *imagining* that it was alcoholic, when it wasn't! In a way, he'd been given *permission* to go into the "high" state, from the drink he'd been offered. And this permission was all he really needed, to start getting "high"!

Similarly, this method gives you the *permission* to go into the "high state," by drinking lots of fruity drinks that taste *similar* to alcoholic beverages, but really aren't!

Books from the internet that show you how to fix many fruity, alcohol-like drinks are:

Drinks Without Alcohol, by Jane Brandt

Non-Alcoholic Drinks to Die For, by Drew Liddle

The Ultimate Party Drink Book, by Bruce Weinstein

Fruit-Infused Water, by Grace Bell

Fruit-Infused Water: 125 Delicious Recipes, by David Lawson

How to Make Your Own Drinks, by Susy Atkins

These are only a few of the many books available on the internet.

In these books are numerous recipes for putting together a tremendous number of alcohol-like drinks that (in reality) contain *zero* alcohol!

Non-alcoholic wine or beer can be added to these drinks. Also a *very small amount* of genuine wine, beer, or hard liquor can be added, if your goal is to drink *less* alcohol, while pretending to yourself to be drinking *more* (as you give yourself *permission* to still get tremendously "high").

So, get some of these books, check out all the recipes for "alcohol mimicking drinks" to make, and give it a go. Perhaps this method can be combined with another method in this book, for example Method #15 (Switch to Marijuana.) As you use the marijuana to get your "high," guzzle down numerous fruity non-alcoholic drinks (with non-alcoholic wine in them?) to satisfy your thirsty "taste for booze"! Try it!

Method #17 - Passionate Hobby

Is there some hobby, sport, activity, or pastime that you really, really enjoy? Or maybe even several of them? Almost everyone derives immense enjoyment and pleasure from *something*, whatever it is!

For me, it's extreme competition. I greatly enjoy chess, bridge, tennis, golf, bowling, ping pong, backgammon, croquet, volleyball, handball, computer games, shogi (Japanese chess), several card games, pocket billiards, and gambling (for small stakes). I love the excitement, adventure, and drama of win-or-lose situations, where you *must* operate at-your-very-best, to win! It really does it, for me!

For you, it's likely something else. But whatever it is, *that's* what can substitute for alcohol! Whenever you crave a drink, do your "ecstatic hobby," instead! Or even have *several* hobbies you love, so that whenever you crave alcohol, you'll have an *entire menu* to choose from, in place of booze.

Perhaps it's not "all-or-nothing" here. As you switch to your favorite hobby, drink only half of the booze that you would normally be drinking. Then, with a compromise of half-hobby (to feel good) and half-booze (to feel good), it will still mean that you've reduced your toxic alcohol intake by 50%! That's very significant!

Also, often people drink alcohol because they feel bad. Well, by starting up again several hobbies you love, you'll start to feel good again, because of the immense enjoyment from your hobbies. As you begin to feel much better, deliberately cut down on alcohol intake, because it's simply no longer needed. Perhaps your drinking will at first reduce by 1/4. Then by 1/2. And then, down to even less. Try it!

To Sum Up: Begin the process of getting your happiness-in-life from your favorite hobbies instead of from booze. Make the switch!

Method #18 - "Why Do I Drink?" Method

Have you ever wondered *why* (deep down) you *really* drink? I'm not talking about the obvious surface reasons: (1) It makes me feel good," (2) "It relaxes me," (3) "It makes me feel more social, with all my buddies, who drink too," (4) "It gives me the guts to approach the opposite sex," (5) "It stops my depression," (6) "It helps me get to sleep," (7) "It's just a habit, which is hard to break," (8) "It helps me unwind from work," etc.

No, I"m referring to the deep, ultra-core reason why you *really* drink. See, you're no dummy! You *know* that alcohol is *poison*! And you've heard "a zillion times" about all the severe health problems that are eventually caused by prolonged heavy drinking. Right?

So, why do you *really* drink? See, the previous eight surface reasons I mentioned have *better* solutions than alcohol. And you know this! Right? Also, you probably sense that, deep down in the *core* of yourself, at the *subconscious level*, there's a totally different and perhaps *repressed* reason *why* you drink

Do you want to die? Are you "burnt out" from the stress or meaningless of life? Are you desperate for love, camaraderie, or significant connection, but getting almost none? Are you suicidally *bored* to death? Is *apathy* the reason, in your very non-exciting, non-adventurous life? Are you in a *rut* and can't see how to get out? Are you in despair from divorce, getting fired, in the wrong job, losing a loved one, bad health problems, money crisis or bankruptcy, old-age problems, or other crisis? Are you lacking, or missing some kind of possible "mission" to help people close to you, help a certain group of people, help animals, or help any other aspect or segment of your world? Or, from some or all of this, do you simply have an overwhelming urge to just give up?

Well, the world is quite a "ball-buster." That's why we have the slogan, "Life's a bitch and then you die." Or, "Life's a rat race." Or, "You can't win for losing." Or, "Shit happens." Or, "Murphy's Law: Whatever can go wrong, will go wrong." Or, "SNAFU: **S**ituation **N**ormal, **A**ll **F**ouled **U**p." Or, "The best-laid plans of mice and men often go astray." Or even, "America's a narcissistic and sociopathic society."

Rarely do we take anyone seriously who claims that "Life's a bowl of cherries," or that we should "Pull ourselves up by our own boot-straps," etc.

Okay, so yes, most of your problems *are* real! Because the world *is* a very problematic and imperfect place! In fact, city life is like a "concrete jungle." So, with your brains, determination, courage, social skills, talents, energy, and all your other positive attributes, you *definitely* need to solve most of your problems and issues in *the best way you can*! Absolutely! (And perhaps even *a little* alcohol can work here, if you can control the urge to drink more and more, and eventually too much, to then destroy yourself!)

But mainly, you need to use all your *strengths* (whatever they are) to deal with *problems* (whatever they are) as best you can, in this chaotic, irrational, imperfect world. As you do this, to create a life as happy and successful as possible, *leave alcohol out of the equation*, because it just makes things worse.

You know this. So apply it! Deal with your life issues by applying your strengths, instead of "copping out" with alcohol! And, you also can keep in mind, "Don't sweat the small stuff," and, "It's all small stuff."

Conclusion: Get in touch with the deepest, core-level (soul level?), darkest reason why you drink, be horrified (shocked) by how you're *destroying yourself*, then begin a *healthy program* of using your strengths to deal with problems, *without any more poison alcohol*!

Method #19 - Reward Method

The essence of this method is to lavishly *reward* yourself with *whatever you've always wanted* (within reason) whenever you're willing to pass up a drink.

The alternative is to give yourself the reward if you only drink a *certain limited amount* of alcohol today. (This limit is the normal amount of alcohol that people ordinarily drink, that is considered healthy, and is decided upon by you beforehand. Often, what is stated as healthy is, one drink per day for adult women, and two drinks per day for adult men. One drink is defined as: 5 ounces of wine, 12 ounces of beer, or, 1 ounce of distilled alcohol "hard liquor").

What do you really like to do? What have you always wanted? Sex? Travel? Delicious snacks or food? Adventure? Doing your favorite hobbies or pass-times? Close camaraderie with others? Love? Parties? Weird experiences of one kind or another? Something else?

Make a list of the top one-hundred things you want to do. It may take an hour or so to do this. Make the time! Then, prioritize your list, numbering everything from 1 to 100, based on how much enjoyment you would get from doing that particular activity. Number One would be the item that you think would give you the most pleasure."

Or else, give everything on your list "Pleasure Points." The most-enjoyable activities would get ten pleasure points, and other activities would get 9, 8, 7, etc., down to 1. Then, every time you pass up a drink, *reward* yourself with ten pleasure points! Immediately cash-in the points by doing pleasurable things on your list, corresponding to the points you just earned and rewarded yourself with. Keep doing this throughout the day, doing pleasurable activities that you *reward* yourself with after passing up a drink!

You'll need to work out the details of this Reward-Point System, tailoring it to your own unique self. But it should result in at least a 50% reduction in toxic alcohol consumption by you, as you "trade in" drinking, about half the time, for the pleasure of doing something you really like (on your list), instead!

Sum-Up: Reward yourself often with "Pleasure Points," by choosing to substitute a pleasure-from-your-list for an alcoholic drink.

Soon your *life* will be filled with much more pleasure, and significantly less booze-drinking! Try it!

Method #20 - Past-Life Ally Teamwork

Of course, it's *controversial* whether we've had past lives or not. Some people think we've had past lives, and other people think we haven't. But it doesn't really matter (as you shall see) for this method to *still work*!

When I took a "Past Lives Workshop" in 1980, I was first guided to enter the hypnotic state. Then, with the right, skillful words, I was told to go back in time and experience a "past life." My subconscious mind cooperated with the hypnotist (it usually does), and eventually I awakened with a *past-life memory* (which was either "real," or "subconsciously created," and perhaps was just to please the hypnotist).

I went through this process several times until I had *ten* past-life memories. These memories *seemed* authentic, since each past-life memory dovetailed with a facet of my personality. But it's very possible that my subconscious mind *created* the ten "past lives" by deliberately making up a past life that closely corresponded to each of these facets of my personality. Why not?

But the reason it *doesn't matter* whether the past-life memories are "real," or "subconsciously made up," is because, either way, the "*you*" in the past life is an "*Ally*"!

Now, what do I mean with this word "Ally"? I first read this word in Carlos Castaneda's books on "Don Juan." It meant an *autonomous force* inside our psyche or mind, similar to a Jungian archetype, or sub-personality, or "alter-ego," or even "inner daemon," that *can* act as a helper, or ally, to a person's ego. Christians would use the "Jesus archetype," here, for example. Buddhists would use the "Buddha archetype." Hindus would use one of several Indian deities, which are all archetypes/allies. Actually, *any mythological figure* (all of which are archetypes) can be used as your Ally! Even in Freudian psychology, either the "Id" or the "Superego" *can* serve as an "ally" to a person's ego (at times). Often of course, we hear about the Id or Superego working *against* the ego, but I've also personally experienced the Id or Superego sometimes being an "*Ally*" to *my* ego!

The goal of this method, obviously, is to encourage and induce an "*Inner Force in You*," or *Ally*, to team up with your ego to *help your ego stop alcohol*!

So, how do you discover this "Inner Force" or Ally? One way is to reflect deeply on which past era or country you're most-*fascinated* with. In your mind, reflect on the past eras in America before you were born: the World War II years, the Great Depression era, the Roaring 20's, the World War I years, the Victorian era, the Wild West era, the Civil War era, the early 1800's, the Revolutionary War years, Colonial times, etc. Then, do this "reflection on past historical eras" for *every country in the world*. Let your "daydreamy imagination" run wild! Chances are, eventually, that you'll find that some past era, in some country, holds the *most fascination* for you! Well, this is where you either (1) definitely had a past life, or (2) have so much "*cerebral voltage*" in your subconscious that an *Ally* can be *created* from this place and time. Actually, the Ally already exists for this past era! It's just that you're finally getting in touch with and *activating* this powerful, potentially ego-helping ally! And remember, *any mythological figure* that you especially resonate with can be your Ally here, too!

The rest is straightforward: Give the ally a name. Draw the ally's picture, with colored pencils, pens, or crayons (or just make a doodle with a regular pen, perhaps). Hold the ally's picture before you, as you talk to the ally. Tell the ally what you want (to help your ego stop alcohol). Ask the ally what *it* wants, in exchange for its help. *Be sure* you're willing to give the ally what it wants (without any double-crossing) afterwards, if the ally *really does* succeed in helping your ego stop alcohol. Then, team up with the ally—let your ego team up with the ally—stop the alcohol, and give the ally what you agreed to give it. *Success!* (Just be *very sure* that you give the ally what it wants, as you agreed, or you may now have an even bigger problem than your alcohol). Remember, absolutely *no double-crossing!*

Method #21 - Subliminal Messages Technique

Subliminal advertising has been found to be very effective, psychologically. Subtle, little, semi-hidden, specially worded messages (that are often ignored by the conscious mind) can still greatly influence the *subconscious* mind! In fact, because of this, subliminal advertising has been *banned* in some places due to its insidious power!

Well, this method will harness the power of subliminal advertising for you to *stop alcohol*! First, you will make up lots of little "stop alcohol" messages and slogans, to post all over your living space. Initially, your conscious mind will notice all the messages everywhere, since they'll seem weird and really stand out. But, as the days pass, the novelty of the messages will fade out, until all these messages just become part of the *background* (of your possessions and surrounding living space). This is when they'll start to *subliminally* work on your subconscious! Every day, and every where, all these versions of "stop alcohol" messages will *insidiously* influence your subconscious mind, in their subliminal manner! And then gradually your desire to consume alcohol will become less and less, until either you stop alcohol or, at least, cut way down!

The "stop alcohol" messages can be written on 3 x 5 cards, in several different colors, to be scotch-taped up, *everywhere*! Half can be printed, and half can be in handwriting script. Put most of them in locations you *view a lot* : refrigerator, kitchen table and sink, bathroom mirror and shower door, on the wall to be seen when sitting on the toilet, on the back of every door, on alarm clock, on cupboard doors, etc.

Here are twenty suggestions, for these worded messages:

Stop Drinking!

You'll die a drunk if you don't stop!

Cut out the booze, *God Damn It*!

Fucking stop drinking already!

You want booze to kill you?

Knock off the booze, *NOW*!

Cut way down on drinking!

Do you want to die from alcohol?

Why do you drink so much? Stop!

Alcohol is a slow death! Stop drinking it!

End your sick booze trip, *Damn It*!

Switch from booze, to something healthier!

Fucking cut out the booze!

Stop alcohol already!

Kick your booze habit, *NOW*!

Shitcan the alcohol addiction, *PRONTO*!

STOP NOW, before booze kills you!

Please stop the alcohol, BEFORE you die.

Let's cut it back, to only *6 beers a day*. Okay?

Stop the booze now, before it's too late!

Obviously, instead of posting *my* messages and slogans, you can *create your own*, instead. Be creative! Perhaps come up with a different, new saying every day. Try it!

P.S. If you're bi-lingual or even tri-lingual, then write these messages in the other language(s) you know, too!

Method #22 - Near-Beer Guzzling

This method is designed to make yourself *sick*, on near-beer and/or non-alcoholic wine. You'll guzzle and guzzle them, forcing yourself to drink more and more of them, until you vomit them up! Then, you'll continue to guzzle even more, on and on, until you throw up again! And on and on, and on! Until you *condition yourself* to associate the taste and smell and sight of alcohol with being sick and throwing up! (Actually, it might be possible to mix in a *very little bit* of real booze here, with the fake booze that you drink.)

What will be needed here also is a cup full of *real* beer, a cup full of *real* wine, and a cup full of your favorite (*real*) hard liquor, placed on a table where you can *intensely smell and tongue-taste them*, as you guzzle the near-beer and non-alcoholic wine. Keep putting first your nose and then your tongue into the three cups of real booze! Then you'll be *very strongly* smelling and tongue-tasting the *real* booze, as you chug-a-lug the fake booze.

If you tried guzzling *real* booze here, instead of *fake* booze, you might *kill yourself* or greatly harm your health from alcohol poisoning, as well as a *super-massive hangover*. So, stick to guzzling the *fake* booze, instead, while just *intensely smelling and tongue-tasting* the *real* booze in the three cups.

Act like you're getting "shit-faced drunk," as you guzzle the fake booze, while dipping your nose and tongue into the three cups of *real* booze. Adopt the mindset that the *fake* booze is the "real thing," helping to convince yourself of this by the intense smelling and tongue-tasting of the cups of *real* booze.

Right behind each cup of real booze, place the bottle that they were poured from. Then as you keep dipping your nose and tongue into the cups of real booze, *strongly stare* at the bottles sitting behind the cups, so that by *sight, too,* you'll be associating the *real* booze with the *fake* booze that you're guzzling! Also, "fondle" the bottle behind each cup, and lift it up and gently tap it on the table, to get your *sense of touch* involved in the process here, too.

Really get into this, with an "I'm gonna get shit-faced drunk" mindset! Guzzle deeply, dip your nose and tongue into the cups, and strongly stare at the bottles of real booze behind the cups, as you fondle the bottles.

Also, go ahead and sing your favorite drinking songs, as you do all this! Maybe: "There is a tavern in the town, in the town." Or, "Roll out the barrel, roll out the barrel of fun." Do a search on the internet for drinking songs, then you can sing all your favorites, as you even sort of pretend to "drunkenly slur the words." (Of course, instead of singing, you could play recordings of these drinking songs.) With this, you even involve your sense of *hearing* in this process, so that: smell, taste, sight, touch, and even hearing are all involved!

Actually, it's fairly important to involve *all five senses* to achieve a total, *ultra-complete* conditioning!

What you're doing is to condition yourself, and *even to sort of* "brainwash" *yourself* (using all five of your senses) with the *association* of alcohol and nauseating sickness! That's why you keep dipping your nose and tongue into the cups of real booze, as you strongly stare at the bottles behind the cups, then fondle the bottles, while you sing or play drinking songs, as you guzzle and guzzle the fake booze, until you throw up, then keep doing this until you throw up again! (Note: If guzzling lots of fake booze *doesn't* make you ever vomit, then *inducing vomiting* by other means may be necessary, like kneeling before a toilet and doing the "heaving" motion, as you smell your own feces, or pressing the back of your tongue with a finger.

The goal of this (strange) method is to make you so ultra-sick of alcohol that you'll never drink again! So, try it!

P.S. If the healthiness of your digestive organs is already not so good, you may need to pass on this method, to avoid serious digestive organ injury from all the vomiting.

Method #23 - Fake Booze While Smelling the Real

If the previous method (of guzzling fake booze until you throw up) is too extreme for you, that's okay. Instead, you can try this *variant*, which will still help you to cut way down on your drinking!

(1) Drink "near-beer" extensively, but *not* to the point of vomiting. As you drink the *fake* beer, keep dipping your nose and tongue into a cup of *real* beer, and stare strongly at the (real) beer bottle placed right behind the cup, as you fondle the bottle. Thus, by smell, taste, sight, and touch, you be experiencing *real* beer, as you chug-a-lug the fake beer. Then as you've sort of had your fill guzzling the *fake* beer, actually drink the cup of real beer (from in front of you on the table). This way, you've *cut way down* on your alcohol consumption by "stuffing" yourself with *fake* beer, before you finish up with only one cup of *real* beer, Try it! This "regimen" really might satisfy your alcohol cravings, yet result in only about 1/4 of *real* beer actually consumed!

(2) Drink non-alcoholic wine extensively, but (again) *not* to the point of vomiting. Follow the strategy above (but with non-alcoholic, *fake* wine instead). You'll drink the cup of *real*

wine at the end, using this "regimen" to cut down your *real* wine consumption to about one-fourth.

This Method #23 can be combined with Method #15 (Switch to Marijuana.) Then you'll get your "high" from the marijuana and one-fourth of the alcohol, but get your taste, smell, sight, and touch *"alcohol-drinking-orgy satisfaction"* from the abundant guzzling of either the near-beer or the non-alcoholic wine! It'll be up to you where to include the pot-smoking with all this. Experiment, to see what works best!

Method #24 - Alternative Drug-High

In this method, you'll be doing (each day) some drug or "high-producing" substance (or method) other than booze!

First of all, for those willing to flirt with *risk and danger*, on your "alternative menu" can be marijuana, cocaine (or crack), heroin (sniffed only), opium, and perhaps even a small amount of ice.

Also included can be LSD, mescaline, peyote buttons, psilocybin mushrooms, ecstasy, and Quaaludes (but not PCP, speed, or strychnine, which are really, really bad for your health). (Interestingly, there are some people who think that the alcoholic beverage companies coerced the United States government to outlaw LSD because so many psychologists and psychiatrists were curing people of alcoholism by using it, in the course of counseling their patients.)

Vast amounts of *caffeine* (coffee, tea, guarana, energy drinks and doses, caffeine pills) can be consumed some days instead of alcohol.

Huge amounts of *sweets* (foods and drinks with sugar, honey, agave nectar, stevia, desserts you especially like) can be eaten, on some days, rather than alcohol. (Consider barfing them up, afterward.)

Great amounts of *salty foods* (chips, popcorn, sushi with lots of soy sauce, etc.) can be substituted on other days, for alcohol.

Exorbitant amounts of *spicy foods* can be consumed on still other days as a replacement for alcohol.

Incredible amounts of your *favorite foods* or desserts can be stuffed and stuffed, even if it results in a little bulimia!

Legal, high-producing herbs can be substituted for alcohol. These include San Pedro cactus (loaded with mescaline), yohimbe, nutmeg, Hawaiian baby woodrose, damiana, Acorus Calamus (sweet flag root, or "rat root"), etc. All these can be looked up on the internet, along with an internet search on "herbs high-producing".

There's a booklet on the internet: "Getting High Legally" that gives instructions on preparation and dose, etc.

Antidepressants such as Prosac, St. John's wort, Valium, or other legal herbs and drugs, can be tried on still other days, instead of booze. Perhaps take *a lot* of them, since you'll just be doing them only one day per month (see below).

"High-producing activities," such as bungee-jumping, sky-diving, (low-stakes) gambling, scuba-diving, high-speed driving, motorcycling, skateboarding, water skiing, paintball competitions, wrestling with friends, competitive tournaments for archery or handguns, carnival rides, motor-boating, flying airplanes, walking at night in semi-dangerous neighborhoods, travel to challenging locations, horror movies, picking up or seducing sexual partners, can strategically replace a day of drinking booze.

Basically, you *compile* a personal "menu" of thirty-one high-producing activities, high-producing "trips" that you can do, instead of booze, *and to distract yourself from booze*, for the day.

You'll need 31 of these "trips," so that you can do a *different one* for each day of every month! (With less than 31, you'll possibly get *bored*—or *addicted*—if any of these activities have to be repeated more than once per month),

Even better is a list of 62, so that you won't have to repeat any "high-producing" activity for two whole months.

Every day, distract yourself from booze with one of your 31 "trips," or high-producing activities. Thus, every day, you'll still be getting your "*high*," but in a different way than from booze! This will save your liver, kidneys, heart, and health from the poison of booze. And since any toxicity from your "list of 31" will hit you only *once a month*, it shouldn't overly harm you *nearly* as much as your daily booze regimen did!

If there are any other "high-producing" activities you can think of (but that I neglected to list), then by all means *include these in your list* (if they really work for you to get your "high" from them instead of from booze).

To sum-up: Totally let your "shadow-side" or "Id" or "Hyde-side" out, instead of drinking alcohol. But do it in a reasonably safe way, to not wreck your life!

Create a super-exciting, thrilling, ultra-high life, from doing one of your 31 menu "highs" each day! Then, at each day's end, feel great that you've gone the whole day without booze. At which point *maybe* you can allow yourself just *one* drink, in celebration (but only if this won't *corrupt you* right back into alcoholism again!)

Method #25 - Crying Out Sadness

When babies feel bad, they cry. Children, too. It's a *natural reaction* to feeling bad. In fact, with babies and children, crying is *almost automatic*! Then, after crying has gone on for awhile, the person feels *much better*! This is because the "crying mechanism" has released the sadness and stress, so that the person feels "relatively okay" again.

The need for *crying*, to deal with sadness and stress is almost like the need for *sleep*, to deal with fatigue and exhaustion (at the day's end). That's how natural and *needed* it is, to cry!

Enter our American Culture's rules, and the "social taboo" against crying (along with taboos against expressing practically *any* other "negative" emotions in public). Of course, it's *especially* taboo for men to cry, but the taboo extends to women significantly, too. No wonder we Americans are so *emotionally blocked* (and emotionally unhealthy)! When emotions are repressed, they don't just "magically" go away. No! Instead, all those "negative" emotions stressfully *build up inside* a person, to cause great inner sadness, depression and despair, along with fear, worry, anxiety, rage, hate, angst, etc. Which is often why we reach for the bottle! Alcohol numbs all these "negative" emotions, but unfortunately the bad health consequences are just too great!

Now, obviously we can't let loose our crying *in public*, because the taboo against it is just too strong, and our life would be seriously compromised if we stopped putting on our best social act (which usually includes a nice smile on our face).

But this certainly doesn't preclude *crying at home alone*, if necessary under the bedding to muffle the sound (so those in next-door apartments and houses won't hear us). Alternatively, we can cry in the shower stall, with the full-blast water sound muffling us. Or, if at work, we can go to the restroom and *secretly* cry a bit (in one of the stalls). This latter option might necessitate the practice of "soundless crying," which is a slightly *advanced practice* involving totally relaxing the vocal cords when crying, so that only a lot of "breathing sounds" are heard.

Most women reading this will have had first-hand experience in the *benefits of crying* to greatly reduce "negative" emotion and stress. In fact, the majority of women are probably *already crying* when necessary, and they may know "secret" and hidden ways to do this without any unwanted consequences in our society (that taboos crying).

It's usually men who haven't cried at all for years (and even decades), and have even *forgotten how to cry*, so that sadness and stress make them automatically "reach for the bottle," instead!

The way to get yourself "sort of" crying again is to:

(1) Give yourself permission to cry again (due to its naturalness and *healthiness*),

(2) *Try* to cry again, by mimicking the breathing, quivering, and facial expressions of crying. Hyperventilating helps greatly to loosen up the "negative" emotions, so that you can attempt to cry them out.

(3) In fact, focus your thoughts and emotions on the awful thing (or things) you want to cry out.

(4) Just keep up this "practicing of crying," and you'll gradually get better and better at crying out your sadness, stress, and angst, instead of reading for alcohol.

(5) Cry under the bed coverings to hide the sound, if necessary (or in the shower). Later on, *soundless crying* can be achieved by *totally relaxing* your vocal chords as you cry, so that just a lot of "heavy breath" is heard, instead of any "wail."

Just keep at it, with lots of practice! Keep remembering that crying is *far* better for you than drinking alcohol!

P.S. You're not at all "weak" if you cry alone, secretly. Instead, you're being *healthy*.

P.P.S. If you are *really blocked* from crying, and think you "can't cry" anymore, check out *Mini-Method #23: Reichian Therapy*, later in this book.

Method #26 - "Brainwashing" Yourself to Not Drink

This method may sound *very extreme*, but your alcohol is causing you so much suffering and *pure hell* that you may consider visiting a "second hell realm" (of self-brainwashing) via a 5-minute daily session, for perhaps one week. By doing this, you'll cure yourself of your hellish alcohol addiction, which otherwise could last your whole life, until it kills you!

Self-brainwashing to stop alcohol is admittedly *not for the timid*, but if it does the job, and if you've "got what it takes" to *ramrod* this brainwashing method into your psyche, well then, your alcohol will stop!

In the Korean War, in the early 1950s, the North Koreans used *brainwashing* on captured American soldiers. By use of extreme pain and torture, over long periods of time, the soldiers' "ego defenses" were gradually broken down until these soldiers were then "opened up" to the propaganda-like "suggestions" of their North Korean captors! Basically, political ideas that "North Korea is good" and "America is bad" were *verbally blasted* at these ego-defenseless soldiers. Eventually, many of these American soldiers were brainwashed enough for the North Koreans to *film* them, with the soldiers on film repeating, "North Korea is good" and "America is bad." In other words, the "brainwashing by extreme, prolonged pain" method *worked*, and people in the United States were rather *shocked* to see this film that North Korea proudly displayed to America.

A similar example, although *much* less extreme, perhaps "semi-brainwashing," occurred in various so-called "empowerment seminars" in America in the 1970s and afterwards. Verbally skilled men called "trainers" would stand in front of a "captive" audience and shout at them (for hours!) that they were "assholes," or "turkeys," or "incompetents" for lazily mis-managing their lives. These audiences were forbidden to leave their painful, hard-backed seats (sometimes not even to take bathroom breaks for long periods) in these marathon, three-day-weekend "trainer-shouting-at-the-audience" ordeals. The goal was to make them "*get it*" that they were each "totally responsible for the quality of their life" and to "stop acting like *victims* by blaming others," because only by "using willpower to be '*at cause*' in their life" would they get the "*effect*" they sought: a successful, happy life.

Four friends of mine took these seminars, told me that the seminars "changed their life," and had considerably more willpower (well, certainly for at least about six months, or until it "fizzled out"). Three other friends also took these seminars and told me that the seminars had little or no effect on them. Still, this is a success rate of over 50%! Thus, even this "semi-brainwashing" seems to often work!

An old movie, *The Manchurian Candidate*, deals with the brainwashing of a captured American soldier. He first is led to think that various suggested hallucinations are real, and then later, he assassinates an American political figure after returning to America. This last episode reminds one of a type of "*post-hypnotic suggestion*" implanted deep in the soldier's mind, by the brainwashing, to later take effect.

Okay, so "enough theory already," the reader may be thinking, about now. And, "How does this self-brainwashing method work?" and "Do I really want to do it on myself?" are probably in your mind, about now. "Get to the point, already!" is probably desired, here now. *Okay! Here it is*:

HOW TO SELF-BRAINWASH YOURSELF

TO STOP ALCOHOL

1) Make a list of things you especially *hate*, and which will cause you to feel "*tortured by repetition*" if you experience them over a long period of time.

2) Weed out from this list (with a red "x" through it) anything that could cause you any physical, emotional, or psychological *damage* (because we certainly *don't* want that to occur).

3) For example, what I *hate* are:

(a) A phone ringing over and over without ever being answered

(b) The sound of a baby crying on and on and on. And on!

(c) Loud barking dog sounds that just won't stop

(d) The smell of feces, urine, or other awful smells

(e) Somebody shouting insults at me (especially if they're true)

(f) My fingers, hands, arms, toes, feet, legs, or body twisted or stretched into painful positions, and held there awhile

(g) Repeated dunking of my head in water (waterboarding?)

(h) A cup of cold water thrown in my face, again and again. And again!

(i) Someone in a swimming pool repeatedly splashing me in the face

(j) Changing a flat tire on a car

(k) Doing yard work

(l) Cleaning anything in the house

(m) Getting really dirty by rolling or rubbing bodily in the dirt

(n) Getting whacked by a *small* stick (even if lightly) over and over

(o) Eating what I hate: eggplant, rhubarb, Brussels sprouts, etc.

(p) Getting "stood up" by someone I planned to meet somewhere, and having to futilely wait and wait and wait!

Enough! You get the idea, here!

4) Now, create your *own* list of all the things that you particularly *hate*! After you finish the list, put a red "x" by anything that you suspect might cause you too much damage (physically, emotionally, or psychologically).

5) Now, record on a tape recorder the "brainwashed suggestion" that you want to *implant into your mind*. It's okay to tape record all of the anti-alcohol statements from Method #2 (Hypnotic Extreme-Disgust Method, starting with "Alcohol is really a *poison*" and ending with "Yes, you'll *stop*, and stop alcohol, right *now*!"). Or you can come up with your *own* "anti-alcohol statements" and "stop-alcohol statements" that could probably be even *more-effective*, since they'll be specially tailored to your own *personal psyche*.

6) Okay, so go through your list of self-tortures in Step (4), and *create a self-torture regimen* that will fill you full of *utter angst* (like a tortured soldier), but won't permanently damage you! You'll need to "feel like hell," yet not be too "messed up" by it, afterward! Perhaps err slightly on the *safe* side here, at first, since you can always "up the anguish" with a "stronger torturous effect" in the future, if the "start-out-milder-torture" doesn't quite do the job!

7) Start the self-torture, feel your angst build and build, then start playing your tape recorder! Experience the hellish pain and angst as you're verbally blasted by an anti-alcohol harangue in your own tape-recorded voice! Or you can directly harangue yourself, or even scream to yourself, about the negatives of alcohol, here, without the tape recorder).

8) It's now up to you to keep *experimenting* with all these brainwashing techniques until you succeed in stopping (or cutting down) your alcohol! Persevere! Learn and get better at it, from each attempted experiment! Congratulations! You've really got *guts*! By doing this, you're definitely *not* one of the timid!

Sum-Up. The *essence* of this method is that the *healthy* "Part A" of you (that wants to end alcohol) is ultra-ultra-fed-up with the *unhealthy* "Part B" of you that *won't* stop (or radically cut back) alcohol! This volcanic, fervently furious fed-upness is so *titanic*, that Part A is even ready to resort to mild brainwashing, semi-brainwashing, or even *full-blown brainwashing* of Part B, to *force* Part B to stop alcohol!

The alternative is an alcohol-wrecked life or death! That's really the choice here: Brainwashing yourself to stop alcohol, or a wrecked life and death! So, when put in this realistic, hard-nosed perspective, this self-brainwashing method isn't at all as "crazy" as it sounds! Especially since the *core* and *inner dynamics* of this method are *routinely employed* by trainers of empowerment seminars and even fast-talking, charismatic, very-effective super-salesmen and -saleswomen! (Yes, very powerful and effectives *sales* can actually be a form of hypnosis and brainwashing. See the book *Hypnotic Marketing* on Amazon.com books.) Also, hypnotic brainwashing can be involved in the strong charm and very effective "spell" that a beautiful (con-woman?) employs on some successful, attractive man that she wants to "win over," to become her husband!

So that's it! A powerful form of hypnosis—brainwashing, and even the combination "hypnotic brainwashing"—are *routinely used* by skillful manipulators, under the innocuous names of "spin," "sales technique," "force of personality," "charisma," or even "feminine wiles." With this in mind, the intention of your "Part A" to brainwash your "Part B" (to stop alcohol) is simply not as "far-fetched" as it sounds! Is it worth a try, perhaps?

You must admit, this is a pretty original method to stop your alcohol. Interested in giving it a shot? (Once again, this method is *not* for the *timid*.)

Method #27 - The "Nine Nega-Emotions" Method

If you've read all the previous methods up to now, you may have noticed how often a *negative emotion* stops-dead your alcohol!

For example, in Method #2 (Hypnotic Extreme Disgust Method), it's extreme *disgust* (from face in spittoon). In Method #6 (6-A-Day Limit), it's extreme *disappointment* (from the limit of 6 not working). In Method #7 (Quit or Die), it's extreme *fear/shock* (from being told by the doctor that you must quit or else die). In Method #8 (The Furious Anger Method), it's extreme *anger/rage/fury*. In Method #18 (Why Do I Drink Method), it's extreme *horror* (from facing the dark, shadowy, ultra-destructive reason why you truly drink). In Method #21 (Subliminal Messages Technique), it's extreme *depression* (from being bombarded by subliminal anti-booze messages). In Method #22 (The Near-Beer Guzzling), it's extreme *nausea*. In Method #25 (Crying Out Sadness), it's extreme *sadness/despair*. In Method #26 (Brainwashing Yourself to not Drink), it's extreme *torturous hate/pain/angst* (from being filled with pain and angst, from the self-torture that you hate).

Well, this method attempts to harness *all nine* of the nega-emotions to stop you from drinking! So that when you're feeling extreme: "disgust-disappointment-fear/shock-anger/rage/fury-horror-depression-nausea-sadness/despair-hate/pain/angst," then you'll finally quit alcohol!

In several books, alcohol/drug addiction is actually compared to *romance*! See, both start out good, with a "honeymoon" of pleasure and "feeling great." Then as "the other shoe drops," and negatives begin to manifest, the pleasure lessens and the pain grows (and grows). Finally (typically), at the end of a romance, all nine of these nega-emotions are so *extreme* that the romance just *has* to end (usually) with a broken heart. It started out so good, yet ended up so bad! Well, alcohol/drug addiction also ends in the same ultra-bad way, and it would be well to "hurry up" this ending process by *deliberately feeling* all nine of these nega-emotions!

Once in ancient feudal Japan, a peasant was grievously insulted in public by a noble, causing the whole village to laugh at the poor peasant. Fervently wanting revenge, the peasant was forced to wait *months* for his chance! So he knew he would have to "keep alive" his vengeance, or it would fade away with time. So the peasant deliberately drank a bitter brew each day, as he renewed his ultra-bitterness towards the offending noble. In this way, his vengeance stayed alive, and eventually the peasant was able to execute his *revenge* against the noble, finally "getting even"!

Similarly, by deliberately feeling daily these nine nega-emotions towards alcohol, you'll fast-forward your "romance with alcohol" to the *last stage of ultra-bitterness*! Then, you'll finally get your "revenge" on alcohol, by quitting it, for good!

In order for this all to work, you'll need something to *trigger* each of the nine nega-emotions towards alcohol, as you feel one nega-emotion after another, towards the booze.

THIS IS WHAT TO DO:

(1) Set up the props and scenario to feel *extreme disgust* towards booze. Perhaps smelling a booze bottle that's been dipped in rotten eggs, urine, dog droppings, badly spoiled food, or the smell from a dead rat, might work. As you look at the booze bottle, and smell its horrid stench, work up as much *extreme disgust* as possible towards booze! The stronger your (felt) emotions, the better! At the peak of your disgust, croak out the words, "*I must stop booze!*"

(2) Set up the props and scenario to feel *extreme disappointment* towards booze. Visualize all the health-wrecking and life-wrecking effects of booze-in-your-life. Really face, fully, what an "awful bummer" booze has been. Emotionally work up the strongest feelings of *extreme disappointment* (towards booze) as possible, here! At the peak of your feelings of nega-emotions, croak out, "*I must stop booze!*" in a voice filled with utter, total angst.

(3) Set up the props and scenario to feel *extreme fear/shock* towards booze. Perhaps you can draw a bottle of booze, then an arrow, then your dead corpse. Then shove this crude drawing in your face and *get* that booze is destroying

and killing you! Really implant the simple message (from your drawing) deeply into your subconscious mind. Because it's true! Booze really is killing and destroying you! As you stare at your simple crude drawing (held so close to your face that it practically suffocates you, perhaps), work up as much extreme fear-shock as possible, at the extreme "in-your-face" *realization* that booze is killing emotion, croak out, "*I must stop booze!*," in a voice of terror, fear and shame.

(4) Set up the props and scenario to feel extreme *anger/rage/fury* towards booze. Perhaps buy a big sack of rice and a metal tennis racket. Spread out your empty booze bottles in plain sight, around the sack of rice (on the floor). Grab the metal tennis racket, and start whacking the sack of rice with it, hard, as you work up enormous volcanic anger/rage/fury/towards booze, and how booze is destroying your life and health and is slowly killing you. Shout and yell here, too! As you whack away, keep building up your anger/rage/fury (towards booze) to higher and higher levels, and at the *peak*, croak out, "*I must stop booze!*" in the most ultra-furious tone of voice that you've ever heard yourself utter! (Be careful that the tennis racket doesn't contact and shatter the glass bottles, which might send glass shards to your eyes and face. Perhaps the glass booze bottles need to be set up *out of reach* of the metal tennis racket, but still very visible to you, throughout.)

(If the noise of all this will bother neighbors, perhaps do it out in the "boonies," in nature. Or drown out your noise with loud rock, punk rock, rap, or drumming music that you play on your stereo in the background. Or do it in a train or subway tunnel, or in your basement or garage. Or do just the racket whacking, with only "muttering" instead of shouting. Or simply hang a rug from a clothesline, and beat it with a broom, in your backyard, which neighbors will consider "normal.")

(5) For *horror*, get what horrifies you the most. Get a picture of your scariest monster, plus perhaps some snakes, big spiders, huge roaches, gila monsters, rats, or gooey snails/slugs. They'll be all made of plastic or rubber, but placed "lighted-up-by-candles and far away from you" (in an otherwise pitch-black room), they'll seem real enough to horrify you. Booze bottles will be placed near or under the "horrifiers." In the dark, work up as much horror as you can towards the booze. At the height of your horror, croak out, "*I must stop booze!*" (Alternatively to all this, you could play a truly horrifying DVD, and surround the DVD set with several booze bottles, to work up the horror feeling towards booze.)

(6) For *depression*, focus mentally and emotionally on all the ways that booze is destroying and killing you, and wrecking your life. Really get into it! Stare at several booze bottles as you do this, and at the very height of your ultra-depression, croak out, "*I must stop booze!*"

(7) For nausea, fill a toilet bowl full of pee or feces, or both. Place empty alcohol bottles in the toilet, amongst the sewage. Kneel in front of the toilet, and start going through the "heaving" motions of throwing up, until you begin to feel *nausea*! When your nausea reaches its peak, stare at the booze bottles in the toilet bowl and croak out, "*I must stop booze!*" (Try to skillfully do this technique without actually throwing up. The goal is to feel extreme nausea, then link up this feeling to booze. The goal is *not* to actually throw up! It's a fine line, here. But if you actually end up throwing up a little, that's okay too. For after all, the goal here is to stop drinking booze by linking nine nega-emotions to booze.)

(8) Cry and/or work up extreme *sadness/despair*. Hold a booze bottle in each hand, staring at them in grief. At the peak of despair, and with both booze bottles right before your eyes, croak out, "*I must stop booze!*"

(9) For hate/pain/angst, review Method #26, and come up with a *mild* torment or torture that brings up enormous hate/pan/angst. Working up the emotion of extreme *hate/pain/angst* to the *max*, and holding (and focusing your eyes on) a booze bottle in each hand, croak out, "*I must stop booze!*"

Sum-Up: The essence of this method is to first work up each of the nine nega-emotions to the max, using suitable props and scenario. The nega-emotion is linked to booze, and at the peak an *anti-alcohol affirmation* is croaked out! You're free to create your own props and scenarios to work up the nine nega-emotions, in your own unique way. Be creative! Also, the anti-alcohol affirmation is *arbitrary*! Perhaps something better than "*I must stop booze!*" can be thought up, by you? Experimenting with various anti-alcohol affirmations may eventually enable you to come up with the best, most powerful words, here. Would "I *stop* booze *now!*" be better? Only by experimenting with various words can you come up with the *most-effective* words, for your own unique situation, here.

This method of combining nine nega-emotions, of extreme intensity, to stop drinking alcohol is *very powerful*. In a way, it's almost like *combining nine of the previous methods!*

Eventually, you might "work out" this method so that it only takes you about 20 minutes to run through the nine nega-emotions. Then, once your booze is stopped, you can run through all this again in just 20 minutes if the urge to resume alcohol starts up again. Instead of a drink, you'll just do 20 minutes of the nine nega-emotions, to totally "kill-off" any re-occurring drinking urge!

Good luck with this method. It might be the very best in this book!

Method #28 - Mesmer's "Animal Magnetism" Method to Stop Alcohol (not hypnosis)

First of all, Animal Magnetism is *not* hypnosis! I will explain why, later, but right away I want to *alert* readers that Animal Magnetism is *totally something else*, which is much more *powerful* than hypnosis!

Many, many people have been quite puzzled by the "Mesmer phenomena" of the late 1700's. How did Mesmer miraculously cure so many people so quickly, of about a dozen different diseases? What exactly is this "Animal Magnetism" that Mesmer claimed he was using?

In order to solve the *puzzle* of Mesmer and Animal Magnetism, I had to read and analyze several books on Mesmer, in order to gather as many "pieces of the puzzle" as possible, to then intuitively flash on the rather extraordinary solution!

These are the most-important clues:

(1) Mesmer repeatedly claimed that he was sending a *physical energy* to his patients. (This energy he called "Animal Magnetism.")

(2) Mesmer claimed that this energy *could not be felt* by *healthy* people, but this energy could only be felt by those who were *sick*.

(3) Mesmer claimed that animals had this energy, and that sick animals could be cured by sending them energy, just as with sick humans. Mesmer's demonstrations of curing horses, cats, dogs, and other sick animals, incidentally, proves conclusively that Mesmer's energy was *not* suggestion or hypnosis, which wouldn't work on animals.

(4) Mesmer claimed dozens of times that his energy was *not* suggestion or some kind of "placebo." In fact, Mesmer became quite angry when anyone would claim that it was "only suggestion."

(5) Mesmer repeatedly claimed that *magnets* were *not* necessary to send his energy! Mesmer only used magnets to aid him sending the energy in his *initial* experiments. But when people began confusing Mesmer's energy with magnetism, Mesmer began to deliberately heal people *without* magnets! Mesmer thus excluded magnets in healing dozens of people and animals, in his later demonstrations.

(6) Photographs of Mesmer obviously show a very physical, earthy, grounded-on-the-earth, sensing, and sensate type of man, who had a lot of physical-type energy.

Now, what is the name of *"life energy"* today, in various parts of the world? In China, it's *"chi."* In Japan, it's *"ki."* In India, it's *"prana."* In Arab countries, the source of this life-force energy is the belly-region, or "hara." In Hawaii, life-force is called "mana." In America, when someone has "healing hands," the healing energy is sometimes called "life force." The movie *Resurrection* tells of a woman who first healed herself, then healed lots of others with this "life force" from her "healing hands." There are several books (on the internet) involving the story of those with "healing hands." There are DVDs to watch of healers in the Philippines, Java, Mexico, and South America who use this "life force" from their "healing hands" to do "psychic surgery," to send electrical current through acupuncture needles, and even to set crumpled newspaper on fire. Martial artists are said to "ground themselves" with this "*chi*" or "life-force." A search on the internet can yield much more about all these different versions of "life-force" energy!

So, Mesmer had "healing hands" and was sending "life force" to his patients through touch (and other methods that he developed). How obvious! in light of all of today's knowledge of a multitude of "life-force technologies."

Incidentally, Brennan, in his book *Occult Reich* (pp.36-38) also figured out that Mesmer's "mysterious force" was *not* hypnosis but was "prana" or "*chi*." The Russians call it "*Bioplasmic Energy*" and have experimented with its use for decades, according to Brennan.

Chinese Medicine, for 6,000 years, has developed several different branches of healing through the use of this "life force," which in Chinese is called "*chi*." Because Chinese Medicine has developed the use of *chi far more* than any other culture (that I know of), I'm going to begin calling "life force" *chi*, for the remainder of this chapter.

The dozen-or-so books I've read on Chinese Medicine say that ordinary, healthy people have plenty of *chi*. It's sick or diseased people who are *chi*-deficient. Also, all these books say that the cause of sickness and disease is simply *lack of chi*!

I once had a girlfriend, whom I'll call Nancy. At the time I was all run-down and fatigued, so daily I used several techniques of Chinese Medicine to re-energize (or re-*chi*) myself. These methods really worked, and I felt my *chi* increasing more and more, every day. But Nancy, in excellent health, did not feel *any chi*-influx, at *all*, from any of my techniques! So, just as Mesmer says, healthy people feel no *chi*-influx, because they're already full of lots of healthy *chi*! But a year later, Nancy had her uterus removed and was chronically fatigued in the hospital after her operation. At this time, I had Nancy try all my *chi*-influx methods once again, and this time, they *all* greatly worked on her! She really felt lots and lots of *chi*-influx. Thus Nancy, when severely deficient in *chi* (after her operation) found that all the *chi* techniques worked great, when she needed them, in the hospital! So, I have had first-hand confirmation of Mesmer's stated principles, both in myself and in my girlfriend Nancy. Also, several other fatigued friends of mine have greatly benefited from these *chi*-influx techniques, too (while healthy friends had utterly no need of them).

There is a technique called *Reiki*, where someone sends energy, or *chi*, to another person with upraised palms. At a booth a a Whole Life Expo in San Francisco, I *actually felt* this *chi* sent to me by the Reiki practitioner at the booth! Several other people told me they felt the *chi* sent by the Reiki method, too. This is similar to Mesmer's statement of sending "*chi*" to people without needing to actually touch them! (Do an internet search on "Reiki" to find out more here, if curious.)

There is a technique called *Deeksha*, where the practitioners put their palms on top of a client's head and send energy/*chi* into their client's brain, to produce happy feelings and even semi-enlightenment experiences. I was in a Deeksha group in Hawaii, where I felt both the happiness and semi-enlightenment, and so did almost everyone else in this group! We would have ecstatic Deeksha celebrations and parties! It works! Perhaps some of the *chi* sent by Mesmer to his clients also went to their brains, to help heal them—not only from physical ailments, but from depression and fear, too. (Do an internet search on "Deeksha" to research this further). But be careful here of sending *too much* palm energy/*chi* to your brain. If your brain starts to feel "overdosed," then immediately stop!

Mesmer was so ridiculed and misunderstood in the late 1700's because "healing hands," "life-force," "*chi*," "Chinese Medicine" (and its 14 meridians of *chi* flowing in the body), "Reiki," "Deeksha," etc., had never been heard of in Europe, where Mesmer lived! Mesmer was *totally on his own*, in an ignorant and skeptical society dominated by quack doctors futilely trying to heal people by bleeding them with leeches! How barbaric! Also, Mesmer's silly name for *chi*, "Animal Magnetism," didn't help much either, since it was confused with both "magnetism" and "animals," which certainly didn't enable anyone to understand much of anything, here!

Thus, Mesmer was the "*Western Father of Chi*" and *not of hypnosis* (or suggestion)!

Chinese Medicine, which is really the *science of chi-influx*, seems to have 16 main branches:

1. *Tonic herbs* (like ginseng) can be brewed and drunk, which gives lots of *chi* to your various organs and bodily parts.

2. *Healing herbs* can be brewed and drunk, to heal over 1,000 illnesses and sicknesses in you.

3. *Acupressure massage* can stimulate the 14 meridians-of-*chi* in you, to abundantly supply *chi* to all your

organs and bodily parts, filling you full of vitality and happiness!

4. *Shiatsu massage* is Japan's excellent version of the above.

5. *Acupuncture* uses tiny needles stuck (painlessly) in key meridian points, to stimulate *chi* and health, exactly in the sick, *chi*-less areas of your body that need it.

6. *Meridian stroking* (of one meridian) sends lots of *chi* to that one specific organ, and meridian stroking of all 14 meridians (one at a time) sends *chi everywhere* in your body, ecstatically!

7. *Jin Shin Do* involves the rapid pressing of about 50 key meridian points, which energizes your body (in just 5 minutes of pressing!).

8. *Chi Gong exercises* (there are many!) get right to the point of filling you up, totally, with maximum *chi*! Do an internet search on "Chi Gong."

9. *T'ai Chi Ch'üan* builds *chi*, and is a great work-out, but it's extremely complex, so that a simplified version of it, *Tai Chi Chih* (do an internet search on a DVD or book about this) is preferable and still works wonders. Alternatively, just slowly "mimicking *T'ai Chi Ch'üan*" by ultra-slow, meditative moving or dancing (along with a *T'ai Chi Ch'üan* DVD; or, just spontaneously) works well, too. Experiment, here, to see what works best for you. Also, try this "meditatively slow moving" in a swimming pool—or even in the ocean—which I call "T'ai-Sea."

10. *Chang energizing* (in Stephen Chang's books, including *The Great Tao*) involves rubbing your hands together vigorously to stimulate *chi*-in-the-hands, then putting these "healing hands" on any part of your body, to heal it. (Avoid the heart and, maybe, the brain.)

11. *Chang* energizing of food or water with *chi*, before eating it, by rubbing hands together vigorously first. Then energize the food or water with "held-over-it" hands, just before eating or drinking it.

12. *Moxa* is also done by acupuncture specialists, and involves drawing toxins and poisons out of the body, with many small "sucking" jar-like containers.

13. *Chi ball manipulation* with hands. Two or three of these metal balls (that emit "gonging" noises) can be circled round-and-round in your left or right hand (or both) to stimulate meridian *chi*.

14. *Chinese foot, hand, or ear massage*, to stimulate meridian *chi*. Ear massage especially brings blissfulness!

15. *Chinese dietary therapy* (of eating all the best *chi-producing* foods, etc.)

16. Any other Chinese medicine techniques that I left out, or that are more *modern discoveries*, like the "acupuncture point clicking device" that can be lined up over any acupuncture point, to greatly stimulate that key point with a loud "click."

Okay! So now you know what to explore (6,000-year-old-*chi*-influx expert's techniques) to maximize your *chi*, health, and happiness! But you can also try borrowing some of *Mesmer's chi* techniques too, from reading his books. You can try combining *chi* with magnets, vats of water (your bath tub?), metallic objects, wands of *chi*, or any other *chi-tools* mentioned in his books. Mesmer was very creative with all of these various *chi*-tools! And you can become so, too. Try inventing your very own *chi-influx tools*, like Mesmer did!

All right already! So what does all this have to do with "stopping alcohol à la Mesmer?" Simply that you can use *all* of these many *chi*-techniques, creatively, to stop your alcohol! (Sorry for the digression, but I needed to *alert* you to the availability of this incredible arsenal of methods from *chi-wise China*!)

When craving alcohol try some *Deeksha* (both un-rubbed together palms on the top of your head) to produce happiness from Deeksha, rather than booze! (If hand-energy on top of your head becomes *too much*, try hands on forehead, or over ears, or one palm on forehead and the other palm over back of your head, visualizing a flow-of-*chi* between them). Drink *abundantly Chang-energized* grape juice, instead of wine. Manipulate 2 or 3 little metal *chi* balls in your hands, to distract you from your urge to drink! Or blissfully massage your ears, to stop the alcohol urge. Stroke the Liver Meridian (and points on it) over and over, and drink a Chinese tea of liver tonic herbs, to heal and strengthen your liver, from all your past alcohol abuse. Etc., etc.!

Sum up: Use all of the best *chi*-influx techniques, from Mesmer (and from China), to get your fix from *chi* instead of *booze*!

Method #29 - Ultra-Powerful Asiatic-Hypnosis Technique

Basically, this method combines the hypnosis in Method #2 (or the self-hypnosis in Method #3) with Method #28's "Animal Magnetism"/*chi*.

The very wise and sly teacher Gurdjieff says several times (in all his books) that there is a much more powerful form of hypnosis in Asia (than the weaker version, which Gurdjieff calls "ordinary European hypnosis"). Gurdjieff also affirms that Mesmer *re-discovered* some of these powerful hypnotic techniques from Asia, in his experiments. But Gurdjieff *never revealed* the secret methods of this ultra-powerful form of hypnosis from Asia (at least not in any of his books, all of which I have thoroughly read).

But the answer is *obvious*, once Mesmer's "Animal Magnetism" is found out to really be Chinese "*chi*." Perhaps (?) one must *fill-to-the-brim* one's *body* with *chi* (from several techniques I mentioned in Method #28). But especially one's *brain* must be (much more carefully) filled with *chi*, without overdosing or harming the (quite fragile) brain. Using "Deeksha," hands can be placed on top of the head, to put "*chi*" into the brain. Be sure to stop this immediately if you feel your brain is being "strained" or "overdosed" with this influx of "hand *chi*"! Those with sensitive brains can put their hands on their foreheads, or over their eyes or ears, or one hand on forehead and the other hand behind the head. Experiment with various hand positions and time lengths, to find out your tolerance, here. Be careful not to strain your brain with too much *chi*! (A headache lasting hours or even days can result from too much *chi* to the brain.) My own first exposure to Deeksha, with 15 minutes of a woman's hand-*chi* to my brain, resulted in a week-long headache! But none of the others in the Deeksha group had this happen to them at all.

All of this is leading to your *maximizing* the amount of (*safe and tolerable*) hand-*chi* into your brain, right before you do Method #2's hypnosis on yourself (or Method #3's self-hypnosis). Thus, filling your brain with hand-*chi* (safely), then doing the hypnosis, will *really* be upgrading "ordinary European hypnosis" to the level Gurdjieff talks about, of "ultra-powerful Asiatic hypnosis"!

It's unclear whether the *body* needs to be filled with *chi*, too (which could make one ultra-restless and less hypnotizable). Maybe *just the brain* needs to be filled with hand-*chi* (safely, without overdosing) before Method #2's hypnosis (or Method #3's self-hypnosis). Maybe everyone is *different* here, and intellectual people need brain *chi*, emotional people need hand *chi* directed into their emotional belly region, and physical people need *chi*-influx all over their body. (All this *chi*-influx would be just before the hypnosis or self-hypnosis starts.)

Lots of experimenting is needed here, by everyone individually on themself. Sorry I don't have all the answers here, but the combining of Animal Magnetism/*chi* with hypnosis is very new, in the West. (But not in the East, according to Gurdjieff.) You could try Method #2 (or #3) and Method #28 by *themselves*, and only *combine* them if that's what really seems *necessary*.

Method #30 - Magic Spell on Yourself, to Stop Alcohol

Many people are quite skeptical about magic, but in this case, when you're doing a spell *on yourself*, it's obvious that it's working very powerfully *psychologically*, and not just through any "magic" forces.

Modern parapsychologists have shown (in abundant experiments) that one person's mind can *influence* another person's mind, at a distance. Even a particular *dream* can be induced in another sleeping person, many studies have shown. Well then, how much more powerful (and believable) it will be, when one part of *you* attempts to influence another part of *you, within the same brain*!

Let's say "Part A" of you wants to stop (or cut down) alcohol, but "Part B" says, "No way!" So, "Part A," out of desperation (due to an alcohol-wrecked life), is resorting to a "Magic-On-Self-Spell," to stop "Part B's" sabotage.

Preparation for the spell: You'll need a ball of white string, scissors, a small table (or cardboard box), a white candle secure in a holder, a full bottle of your favorite booze, and a white bucket, plus a private place to work this spell, at night. Also (most important of all), you'll need a notebook and pen handy, in order to write down solutions in your "magic diary" (notebook) afterwards.

DOING THE MAGIC SPELL:

1) Take off all your clothes, to be in-the-nude. (If you live in a very cold climate, you can be clothed, even though this could render the spell less powerful.) If you wear glasses, it's better to take them off too, unless you really, really need them to see.

2) Use the ball of white string to create a pentagram about 6 to 8 feet in diameter, on the rug or floor. (A pentagram is a 5-pointed star, with a circle going around the 5 tips of the star.) If the lines of white string aren't quite straight or circular, that's okay. If you need to cut the white string into two or more parts to do this, that's okay, too.

3) Place the small table (or cardboard box) at one of the star-tips of your pentagram, with the candle—secure in its candle-holder—sitting in the middle of the table. Light the candle, and turn off the lights, to work in the darkness (to candle light) at night. Make *absolutely sure* that the candle won't fall over and start a fire!

4) The white bucket can be in front of the table (barely within your pentagram), and the opened-but-full bottle of booze can sit on the table (securely, so that it doesn't fall over and spill). Your "magic diary" notebook (with pen handy) can be placed under the table, for now.

5) Stand, nude, in the middle of your pentagram, and do the Lesser Banishing Ritual of the Pentagram (or Rubric Ritual) from Method #4 of this book. But if you don't have much time, you can *skip* the Rubric Ritual and just move-on here, to (6). (This *could* reduce the power of this spell, a bit.)

6) Retrieve the white bucket and opened bottle of booze, then kneel, nude, in the middle of your pentagram, facing the lighted candle. The white bucket is in front of you, and perhaps your non-dominant hand holds the opened bottle of your favorite booze. But really, the bottle of booze needs to be held by the hand

(connecting to the brain-hemisphere) that most likes to drink! Experimentally hold the booze in each hand, to find out which hand is the "drinking hand," here.

7) Now, come up with a name for the "Part A" of yourself that wants to stop alcohol. It could be your first name, preceded by "I." Next, come up with a name for the "Part B" of yourself that *refuses* to stop alcohol. It could be your *middle* name, preceded by "Me." (For the remainder of this spell, I'll use "I, First-name" for your "Part A," and "Me, Middle-name" for your "Part B.")

8) Look in the approximate direction of the candle (without straining your eyes too much). Focus your consciousness and awareness into "Part A" of yourself, and powerfully state "We *must* stop alcohol! It's wrecking our lives! I, First-name, declare that this *must* be *so!*"

9) Now, switch your consciousness and awareness into "Part B" of yourself, as you wiggle the booze bottle in your "drinking hand," and say, "No, I like to drink. Me, Middle-name, says *Fuck You!*" Then take a swig of your favorite booze, and hold it in your mouth, as "Part B" savors the taste of it, but *don't swallow it!*

10) Now switch back to Part A, and vehemently spit the mouthful of booze into the white bucket. Then "hawk" and spit again into the bucket and say, "No! I, First-name say that we *must quit!* Alcohol is wrecking our lives!"

11) Now, switch back to "Part B" and say, "Too bad! Me, Middle-name, is gonna keep drinking!" Take another

swig of booze, and savoringly hold it in your mouth, but without swallowing.

12) Switch back to "Part A," again vehemently spit out the booze, and again "hawk" and spit into the bucket. Then say, "Absolutely not! We *have* to stop drinking or we're *fucked*! I, First-name, say we *MUST STOP*!"

13) At this point, keep on switching back-and-forth from "Part A" to "Part B," as you *enact a drama* of your two sides *arguing it out*! Let any dialogue between them *flow spontaneously*, as they *fervently* debate this crucial alcohol issue, in your life. For the *goal* of all this is to *get them talking and communicating* (however toxically, at first) in order to eventually arrive at a solution of some sort (perhaps a limit of six beers a day?). Obviously, any compromise solution needs to be rigidly adhered to, or it's not really a solution at all, but "bullshit." "Part A" of you may be the Parent/Adult side of you, while "Part B" may be the Adolescent/Child side of you. Thus, "Part A" and Part B" verbally fighting it out (like this) may be similar to verbal battles between parents and teenagers in a family. Therefore, any "solution" may need to be similar to actual, real-life solutions that parents and teenagers arrive at, in actual, real-life family situations!

14) Obviously, this magic ritual needs to end with "Part A" having the *last word*, and with no alcohol actually drunk (only tasted, then spit out). So, at the end, after spitting out the last mouthful, then "hawking" and spitting into the bucket, "Part A" can say (with finality), "I, First-name, declare that alcohol is

forbidden from now on! *Please*, Middle-name, join with me in this! And if you can't stop "cold-turkey," *please* agree with me to do one of the other methods in this book. *Please, please, please*! I beg you, Middle-name. We *must* stop our drinking! And, if you stop with me, I'll give you something else you want, regularly, as long as *that* doesn't wreck our life, too. So please, let's stop. Okay? What do you want, or what other method of stopping shall we try?

15) At this point, just keep kneeling there nude, in front of the candle in the dark room, and allow your intuition to flash on any ideas, feelings, hunches, or sensations. If you want, you can hold your hands together in the "praying" gesture, as you kneel. For it's *these* ideas, feelings, hunches, or sensations that could lead (miraculously) to the "Third Force" solution. See, the First Force is "Part A" of you. And the Second Force is "Part B" of you. Left alone, Forces One and Two just continue to battle it out. So, the goal is to (rather miraculously) get to Third Force: a true, workable solution. It's extremely hard to describe *how* to get to Third Force, but this magic ritual is designed to do *exactly that*: to get to Third Force, which is a solution utterly designed to fit your unique personality, to deal with your alcohol craving issues!

16) Write down any insight, intuition, idea, feeling, sensation, or *anything else* that might help, into a Magic Diary that you start. *Do it immediately*! For often anything after a Magic ritual can fade as quickly as a dream! Wouldn't it be a real shame, if you received (intuitively) the answer to your alcohol

issues, after the ritual, but failed to write it down and then *forgot it*, because you were in too much of a hurry to put everything away and put your clothes back on? No! Take the time, *now*, to write down any *clues* toward the Third Force solution, that are "in your aura" after the Magic ritual. This is the *very most important part* of all this!

17) Put the lights back on, blow out the candle, put your clothes (and glasses?) back on, roll up the string (so no one will stumble across the pentagram and think you're weird), and hide your Magic Diary in a *secret place* (so no one will find out about the magic and be irrationally afraid of you, or gossip about you). Best to put the candle away, too. However, unless it's *absolutely certain* that no one will ever stumble across your "magic room," perhaps because you keep the door to the room *locked*, then you can leave everything out, for convenience in doing this ritual again. And again! And, still again! Until you record enough insights in your Magic Diary, to arrive at Third Force solution, and successfully deal with your alcohol issue in a way that satisfied (relatively) both "Part A" and "Part B" of you!

Good luck with this method, in arriving at your unique *SOLUTION*!

Caution: As I said at the end of Method #4, those with a history of mental problems (or mental illness) may need to *skip* this method! See, your whole life up to now may have been lived with a sort of "wall" (in your brain) between "Part A" and "Part B" of you. (Gurdjieff calls this brain-wall a "buffer," and says that removing mental buffers may be a bit dangerous.)

If, up to now, the success and stability of your life is dependent on "Part A" and "Part B" of you being *separated* by a mental *"buffer,"* then the *possible* removal or even *reduction* of this "buffer" by Method #30 could be ill-advised, perhaps.

How well will "Part A" function at *work* if "Part B" isn't sufficiently "walled off" (mentally) to allow "Part A" to do your job well and not get fired? Will "Part B's" voice continue in your head, arguing and demanding alcohol, well into the next day following this doing of Method #30?

Seriously, are you *mentally together* enough to handle a "temporary merging" of "Part A" and "Part B" as they argue, mediate, and try to (alcoholically) work it out?

Some people can have their "Part A" and "Part B" intensely merge to "work it all out," and be okay afterwards (quickly reverting back to normal). This author is one of those people. Others might take *hours* or even *days* for "Part A" and "Part B" to adequately separate again to allow normal functioning in their life or job!

Actually, *this entire book* deals with the paradoxical problem of "Part A" of you wanting to stop alcohol, and "Part B" insisting on drinking alcohol, *anyway*! Perhaps you need to do another method that allows "Part A" and "Part B" more *distance* (and maintaining the mental buffer between them to insure continued good mental health).

If you think it's too risky to "play around" with the possible removal (or reduction) of the mental *buffer* between "Part A" and "Part B," then maybe instead, you could "role play" parts A and B with a *friend*. Let's call this:

Method #31 – Role-playing Parts A and B with a Friend

First, you're "Part A," as your friend role-plays "Part B," as you argue-out, mediate, and talk out this key "drink-or-not" serious problem, of yours. Then, switch! You be "Part B," as your friend role-plays "Part A." Again attempt a successful talking-of-it-out! Keep switching back and forth, with your friend, for perhaps an hour. Each time you (and your friend) are *either* "Part A" or "Part B," but *never both-at-once*! Thus, your mental buffer will *not* be strained this way, and your life can continue to be successfully lived with "Part A" and "Part B" (opposites) healthily separated by your (needed) mental buffer.

Actually, perhaps you've been a bit *leery* of putting a magic spell on yourself (Method #30) from the start? Okay! Instead, try *this* method. Maybe you and your friend can even try doing it in the dark, to candle light? Anyway, give it a try!

Method #32 - Put Together Your Own Method from Bits and Pieces (from this book)

Obviously, everyone reading this book is *different*. Thus, everyone is going to have a *different attitude* (of either like or dislike) towards *each* of the 55 stop-alcohol techniques!

This method enables you to combine (or team-up) all your *favorite* stop-alcohol techniques into a single, very effective, *system*.

After you've read through all 55 techniques in this book, go back to the table of contents and put a checkmark next to the five stop-alcohol techniques that you like best.

Now, how can you *combine together* all five of these favorite techniques into a workable system? In thinking and analyzing how to do this, feel free to slightly modify any of the 55 techniques to suit you better, in your uniqueness! Perhaps this "combinational thinking" will even enable you to discover some *new* technique derived from this combination of "already-read-about techniques."

This method is for creative people and rebels! It's for those who want to use this book as a springboard, to devise *their own* very individual system, to stop drinking alcohol. Well, go ahead! Devise your own original method, or combination of methods and mini-methods, then implement your unique system, to stop alcohol in *your very own way*! Good luck!

Method #33 - Love Yourself Method

Often people drink alcohol (and do every other bad habit under the sun, too) because they *don't love themselves much*! For, if they truly loved themselves, then they wouldn't be abusing alcohol (or doing all the other bad habits) in the way that they're doing.

But loving yourself is one of the *hardest things to do*, somehow. And few people that I know are doing a very good job of it!

There's a book on Amazon.com entitled *Love Yourself Like Your Life Depends On It*, by Kamal Ravikant. This author's method is basically to say to yourself, "I love myself, I love myself" etc., over and over, hundreds of times a day. It's taking the "saying of affirmations" method to an extreme! But the trouble is, affirmations seem to work a little at first, but then they may work hardly at all. Why is this?

My experience with affirmations is that, within a minute of starting to say an affirmation, I begin to hear a critical voice *in my head* actively saying the opposite! For example , after I say, "I love myself" a few times, I begin to hear "Aw, come on . . . no, you don't . . . what are you saying that crap for . . . you know you don't really love yourself . . . what bullshit! . . . hey, knock it off . . . god-damn-it, knock fucking off that goddamn shit! . . ." etc.

Other people may not have an inner critic that's quite as *active* as my inner critic is, in vehemently trashing affirmations, but they still probably experience *enough inner resistance* to affirmations to eventually *thwart them*, rather effectively. So that the continued repetition of the affirmation begins to feel *futile*, and then becomes *boring*, and then the hollow-sounding affirmation tends to "peter out" and stop! It's simply *not* working!

Well, after decades of reading psychology and self-help books, and actively experimenting on myself with *thousands* of techniques, *I've actually found a way to make affirmations work*! This means that, using my "*Secret To Make Affirmations Work*" technique, you can then use Kamal Ravikant's method (in his book *Love Yourself Like Your Life Depends On It*) and say over and over "I love myself" and actually *finally* become successful in genuinely, truly loving yourself!

Unfortunately, the explanation of my technique is *complicated*, so please bear with me, as the *rewards* of using my technique are *spectacular*, namely that you'll experience *tremendous self-love, finally*! Also, once you *understand* my technique, it's *very easy to do*!

There's a book by Schiffer on Amazon.com entitled *Of Two Minds*. Schiffer is an absolute *genius*, who proves in this book that the two hemispheres in our brain are really *two separate personalities*, which can be called P-1 and P-2. And that, *usually*, the personality of one hemisphere (P-1) is mature and self-loving, but that the personality of the other hemisphere (P-2) is rather immature and troubled (in some way). The mature hemisphere's personality, P-1, is *already in agreement* with the idea of "I love myself," but the troubled hemisphere's personality, P-2, is not in agreement at all with the idea of, "I love myself." Thus, P-1 says, "I love myself," but P-2 verbally *trashes* this idea (for example, "Bullshit!").

Well, there's a way of *inputting into your brain* the idea of "I love myself" by enhancing P-1 while gently blocking off P-2! This is because brain hemispheres P-1 and P-2 look out through our two eyes in a unique way. See, when you look with both eyes to the extreme left (as your head still faces straight ahead), you activate *only one* of your hemispheres, as the other hemisphere is *excluded* from perception (and, perhaps, consciousness). And when you look with both eyes to the extreme right (while keeping your head facing forward), you activate *only the other* of your two hemispheres, as the first one is excluded from perception (and, perhaps, consciousness).

By creating a simple pair of "vision-block glasses," then putting them on, you'll be able to activate brain hemisphere P-1 and exclude brain hemisphere P-2, so that when you say over and over, "I love myself," it will then—finally—*sink in*!

Incidentally, there's a "shortcut" around making these glasses. Instead, when swinging your eyes to the left (without turning head), put your right palm over your right eye, blocking out all light. This activates P-1, only. Then, when swinging your eyes to the right (without turning head), put your left palm over your left eye, blocking out all light. This activates P-2, only. Using your eyes and hands like this is a way around having to create Glasses A and Glasses B, as described below.

Remember though, that P-1 and P-2 are reversed (in left and right) for 50% of all people.

For an example of the finished glasses, see a picture on http://descubrituser.com.ar/wp-content/uploads/2017/01/tic.jpg.

Here is the first pair of vision-block glasses ("Glasses A") to create:

GLASSES-A

1. Obtain a simple, ordinary glasses frame—not reading glasses frame—without lenses.

2. Scotch tape cardboard over the frame's two openings in such a way that your *right* eye's vision is blocked by the cardboard. Also, your *left* eye can only look out of a 1-inch slot at left of the frame's left opening.

Now, create the second pair of vision-block glasses ("Glasses B"):

GLASSES-B

1. Obtain another identical glasses frame.

2. Scotch tape cardboard over the frame's two openings, in such a way that your left eye's vision is blocked by the cardboard. Also, your right ey can only look out of a 1-inch slot of the frame's right opening.

Making these opposite pairs of Schiffer Goggles is thoroughly described in Frederic Schiffer's book *Of Two Minds*.

Amazingly, wearing and looking through Glasses A activates *only* the right hemisphere of the brain, and wearing and looking through Glasses B activates *only* the left hemisphere of the brain! Incredible, right?

Now, put on Glasses A and notice how you feel. If you feel more happy and relaxed, then this is probably P-1, your more-mature hemisphere ("grown-up you"). But if you feel stressed and angry, then this is probably P-2, your more-immature hemisphere ("teenage you"). Start saying to yourself, "I love myself," over and over. If you accept this "I love myself" affirmation, almost naturally, then the brain hemisphere you've activated is probably P-1. But if you criticize, oppose, or angrily want to stop, then you've probably activated P-2.

Now, put on Glasses B and go through the same process as before. If Glasses A activated P-1, then Glasses B should activate P-2. But if Glasses A activated P-2, then Glasses B should activate P-1!

With *this author*, Glasses A activates P-1 and *blocks-off P-2*! Thus, when I wear Glasses A, with a pair of *green color-therapy glasses* over Glasses A, and I say "I love myself" over and over, then *incredibly, I hear no verbal trashing remarks from P-2*! This is because Glasses A (for me) exclude P-2 from the visual field (and consciousness).

Amazingly, when I (psychically) tune-in to what's going on in P-2, *it feels like P-2 isn't even aware that the saying of "I love myself" is going* on!

Then, after maybe ten repetitions of "I love myself" (totally unopposed by P-2), I feel a strong desire to hug myself (by crossing both arms over my chest), so I do this (hug myself). I'm strongly feeling "super," happy, and full of self-love (totally unopposed by P-2, still).

And then, I start to feel the emotions of self-love slowly "percolate" through the corpus callosum (the brain part that can either connect the two hemispheres, or, when stressed or tensed, keep them more-separate). Gradually, feelings of self-love go over to P-2, via my corpus callosum, and start to make P-2 feel a *little* more self-love, in this *indirect manner*! And when I (psychically) tune into P-2, to see what's going on, I find *P-2 doesn't really mind it*! In other words, P-2 vehemently objects to the affirmation "I love myself," but it's actually okay with P-2 if the *feeling of self-love* slowly percolates across the corpus callosum from P-1 to P-2! So that, through this method of using Glasses A, I've (miraculously) actually succeeded in filling myself up with enormous feelings of self-love!

Green color-therapy glasses can be bought on the internet. ColorTherapy.com is a site that works here. Do a search for "color therapy glasses" to get all the sites and the best price, which may be around $15. (Perhaps a few layers of green cellophane, taped over Glasses A or Glasses B, can also work, instead.)

Now, even though with *me*, my left eye (and right brain hemisphere) are P-1, I've found that only *50%* of the people I've experimented on, with Glasses A and Glasses B are the same as me! The other 50% are the *opposite* of me, and Glasses B (activating their right hemisphere) have the key to activating P-1 and blocking P-2's critical resistance to the "I love myself" affirmation.

That's why I had you make *two* pairs of "vision-block" glasses. It's because I didn't know whether Glasses A or Glasses B would work for you, with this "I love myself" affirmation method.

Also, it may be necessary to alternate between Glasses A and Glasses B, back and forth, over and over, for a while, until you can "vibe out" which glasses (A or B) activates P-1 and blocks P-2.

Anyway, when you find out whether Glasses A work, or Glasses B work, then put on the successfully working glasses and start saying lots and lots of "I love myself" affirmations (as described by Kamal Ravikant in his book *Love Yourself Like Your Life Depends On It*). Now that my technique here, which is the "*Secret to Make Affirmations Work*," can be combined with Kamal Ravikant's book, then it is indeed very worthwhile for you to buy and make use of Kamal Ravikant's book!

Note: Affirmations of "I love myself" can be *greatly empowered* by rapidly moving your eyes from side to side, as described by Beaulieu in *Eye Movement Integration Therapy*.

Note: If you do an internet search for "Louise Hay I love myself," you can be introduced to the life-work of this teacher that focused on affirmations and self-love. A simple-to-do technique of hers is to look at yourself directly, with both eyes at the same time, in the mirror, and say, "I love you," every day, or even multiple times every day. Try this with Glasses (A or B) or with green color-therapy glasses worn over them.

So that's it! You now have a technique for finally feeling lots and lots of true, genuine love for yourself, as you hug yourself, feeling absolutely ecstatic! Do it! Often! And very probably it will help you to cut down on alcohol, or even stop alcohol altogether!

P.S. When you've found out which Glasses (A or B) activates P-1, then do *not* wear the opposite pair any more, which stressfully activates P-2, only causing angst.

Another extremely powerful way to love yourself is to build *Temple Grandin's love box*! Buy the DVD: TEMPLE GRANDIN, familiarize yourself with her life story and extraordinary invention of the love box, then build a love box yourself (the blueprint is on the internet) or even buy one. I experimented (very carefully) by wedging my body (*sideways*) between the mattress and box springs of my bed. (Be careful not to hurt your back this way!) I found that this snug, feeling-of-being-hugged experience tremendously increased my self-love. It may have been very similar to the feeling one experiences in Temple Grandin's love box. Indeed, if Temple Grandin's love box really increases your self-love to where you'll give up alcohol and thus save your health and life, then isn't it well-worth-it to build or buy one? Watch the DVD: TEMPLE GRANDIN, then decide!

Still another powerful way to love yourself is to buy four large (4-foot long) teddy bears. When I bought them, they were about $40 each, so your investment might be $160, way less than the cost of buying booze for the rest of your life. Lying down in bed on your right side, position yourself so that your chest is hugging teddy #1, and teddy #2 is hugging the front of your legs. Teddy #3 is behind you, spoon-hugging your back, and teddy #4 is also behind you, spoon-hugging the back of your legs. Thus, you're totally immersed in an "ocean of teddy-bear love," as you're being hugged front and back by the four big teddy bears. You feel so, so loved by this! It really works! Try it! It almost feels like being loved and hugged, front and back, by two lovers at the same time! Or even do Temple Grandin's love box *in combination* with the Glasses (A *or* B, whichever brings out P-1 for you) and say "I love myself." Or, be hugged by the four teddy bears as *simultaneously* you wear the Glasses, and affirm over and over, "I love myself"!

And still one more way of loving yourself is to buy (on the internet) my other book, *Love Yourself: How to Actually Do It!* The methods of self-love in this book will also work exceptionally well to greatly help you to love yourself and give up booze!

So, that's it! You now know how to *effectively* start loving yourself *lots* more, which should greatly help in cutting down or stopping booze. So, go ahead and start doing it. Today!

Method #34 - Stopping Sugar

Because alcohol drinking is often due to *depression*, getting to the *core* reason why we're depressed, and stopping the depression, will stop the booze!

Amazingly enough, *sugar* is really the culprit here. First of all, the processed white powder known as sugar (or *sucrose*) is not really a food at all, but is a *drug* (like cocaine)! That's why this *sucrose* gives its drug-like high! And, like most drugs, it is actually more of a poison, in its harmfulness. Haven't you ever noticed how *different* this strange, artificial white crystalline powder is, from all the other actual, real foods you eat? Unfortunately, we've all been heavily brainwashed by society that sugar (*sucrose*) is "just another food", when it's *not*!

Well, by frequently ingesting this drug *sucrose* (artificial sugar) we greatly enjoy the taste and get our drug-like "sugar-high", but the harmful *sucrose* gradually wrecks our pancreas, liver, and adrenals. This compromises the ability of our body to maintain balanced *glucose* (blood sugar) in our blood stream. (Notice here that artificial *sucrose* and natural *glucose* are utterly different in their effects on us.) Eating *sucrose* (artificial sugar) forces the pancreas to secrete insulin, which then reduces *glucose* (natural sugar in our blood stream), which then causes hypoglycemia (low blood sugar), leading to depression and booze-craving.

This is all explained thoroughly in Dufty's best-selling book "Sugar Blues", especially on pages 86 and 148. Alcoholism, often caused by damaged adrenals, pancreas, and liver, from *sucrose* ingestion, is mentioned on page 72. Reading Dufty's very entertaining book "Sugar Blues" is highly recommended, to thoroughly educate you about all this!

An unnatural junk food diet, along with all the *sucrose*, makes things even worse. Thus, the cure is to stop *sucrose* and eat mostly whole grains and vegetables, which Dufty explains on pages 22-23, and page 105.

Thus, the essence of this method #34 is:

(1)   Read Dufty's book "Sugar Blues" to totally understand why *sucrose* is a harmful *drug* that must be stopped!

(2)   Read my brief 36-page book "Stop Sugar Craving Fast" that gives a quick and easy way to *effortlessly* end all *sucrose* craving (fast).

(3)   Switch to a natural diet of whole grains, vegetables, some fruits, salads, beans, a little fish, miso, and tofu, etc.

(4)   All this will end any hypoglycemia and lead (gradually) to blood *glucose* being balanced and normal again! (Because *sucrose* ingesting will stop wrecking it all.)

(5)   This will result in a *naturally content state* of "feeling good" (ending any depression).

(6)   Then you'll have no need for alcohol, because you already feel good!

Conclusion: If you have the sustained interest to read a very entertaining 234 page book (Dufty's "Sugar Blues"), plus a brief 36 page book (my "Stop Sugar Craving Fast"), to then (effortlessly) stop sugar and (more difficult) change your diet, then you'll feel so great that you'll no longer need alcohol!

But, even if you just stop *sucrose* (only), and eat a *relatively* good diet, this should lead to *much less* alcohol drinking!

Finally, a "shortcut" here is to eat as much organic turmeric powder as you comfortably can with all your meals (2 level teaspoons/meal?) Turmeric greatly stops sugar-craving, plus it has extremely healthy antioxidant power. Be sure to add 1/10 teaspoon of *organic black pepper* to each level teaspoon of turmeric powder, too, plus a small amount of coconut oil. These two will increase the absorption and effectiveness of the turmeric powder enormously.

So,

(1) turmeric greatly reduces sugar-craving.

(2) Little or no sugar greatly reduces hypoglycemia and depression.

(3) Little or no depression then causes little or no alcohol!

Good luck with this method!

P.S. You might need to re-read this method a few more times, to thoroughly understand it all.

23 Mini-Methods That Stop Alcohol

Mini-Method #1 - Ally/Sub-Self Method

No matter how much our society gives us the idea that we are "one," instead, really, we are "many." That is, every one of us has many different parts that can be called "sub-selves," or "sub-personalities," or "characters," or "archetypes" (in Jungian psychology), or "allies" (in the Carlos Castaneda series of "Don Juan" books).

Start off by making a list of all your different parts. You probably have a worker, a player, a social communicator/ actor part, a bossy part, a romantic part, a loyal friend part, an internalized father/mother part (Freud's "Superego"), and a depressed, angry, fearful, upset child part (Freud's "Id"). Also, Jung's archetypes of "Shadow," "Trickster," and "Hero/Warrior/Savior" are probably in the mix, too. Is there also a lazy part, or a goof-off part, along with a comedian? Already that's 14, if you have them all. See what I mean, how ultra-complex we all are?

Now, examine all your sub-selves and find perhaps the *three strongest*, who really want to help you to *stop alcohol*. Perhaps they would be three of these four: the *Superego*, the *Hero/Warrior/Savior*, the *bossy* part, or the *worker*.

So now, when you've chosen your strongest sub-selves, all with strong willpower to help you to stop alcohol, draw all their faces! Using colored pencils or even crayons, use your *intuition* to draw their faces, either on white "card stock" or just on 8-1/2 x 11 printer paper.

If you're new to this "intuitive drawing" or "drawing from your subconscious," take your time. But, try to intuitively "channel" three or four drawings. Take three or four days, or even a week, if you need to.

These three or four drawings of your strongest sub-selves are now your *allies*! And, by talking to, and calling on these allies to help you, they'll often respond to help you stop drinking alcohol!

Call on the *strength* of these allies as you look at their faces that you've drawn. Ask, beseech, or even *command* them to help you! Perhaps say, "All right, already, all you guys! You're the toughest dudes I've got in this psyche of mine! Well, let's stop this darn alcohol problem! Enough, already! Let's have some *power* to *totally knock off* this *alcohol bullshit* that's wrecking our life! Come on! Let's do it, you guys! I know you have the *power* to make it happen, so let's go! Yeah! Let's do it! Now!"

Obviously, everyone will have their own style of talking to their strongest allies. So, do all this in *your own way*! Perhaps, also, these allies can distract you from drinking by getting into *their* favorite activity, instead.

Mini-Method #2 - Cayenne Pepper

Cayenne pepper greatly helps you to stop alcohol! It produces endorphins that help raise mood, similar to the "mood-raising" of alcohol. Cayenne helps overcome, and bring down alcohol cravings.

Very tonifying and healing to the stomach, is cayenne pepper. Gastritis and stomach pain can easily be caused by alcohol over-consumption. This pain and inflammation of the stomach lining can be relieved by cayenne pepper!

Cayenne stimulates the alcohol detox process, by facilitating the excretion of alcohol toxins faster.

You can add a few pinches of cayenne to your glass of water. Or, slowly drink warm water with ¼ teaspoon of cayenne, which is very healthful for the heart.

Don't use cayenne if you have stomach ulcers.

Experiment with a little *organic* cayenne, in your drink or food. You'll be glad you did!

Mini-Method #3 - Depression-Stopping Method

It may all boil down to depression. Many *people drink because they're simply unhappy*! See, a happy person doesn't need to drink much, if at all, because they're already happy! At a party, they may drink some to get "high," but really, they don't *need* to drink. Even a "neutral" person (between happy and sad) doesn't really *need* to drink, because they'll be able to find plenty of enjoyable things in life to do.

So, the problem isn't really *alcohol*. The problem is *depression*! Depression is the *cause*; drinking alcohol is the *effect*. That's why it's so hard (almost impossible?) to stop alcohol (the effect), because you haven't relieved depression (the *cause*)!

Therefore, the whole *solution* to the drinking problem is: How to gradually (or quickly!) switch from a state of unhappiness to a state of more happiness. Or, at least from unhappiness to neutrality. Or, even from unhappiness to a "semi-unhappiness," or a "lesser unhappiness," which can be more-easily tolerated, so that you don't need to reach for alcohol.

In a way, *alcohol is an antidepressant*, although it is an extremely unhealthy one, due to all the harmful-to-health, and harmful-to-life-success, side effects.

Once, someone said to me, "Bars are full of unhappy people." I was surprised at this, at first, because I had experienced so many bars full of laughing, joking, clowning-around people who didn't seem unhappy at all! But, the bar people were like this because of all the *alcohol* they were drinking. They were "drugged"—on beer, wine, and hard liquor—and that's why they seemed so jolly. If they hadn't been unhappy in the first place, they wouldn't have even *needed* to go in the bar, to drink the alcohol. Instead, they would have found plenty of amusing or useful *other* things to do, instead of "bar drinking."

This now *reframes* the whole problem of drinking alcohol. It is simply *unhappiness* and *depression*, enticing a person to take a handy, legal, non-prescription drug (alcohol) to stop the depression. The trouble is, that alcohol over time wrecks your health and life!

Instead, you can reduce your unhappiness with *other solutions* that either don't harm your health, or don't hurt your health anywhere near as much!

Besides taking some anti-depressant herb, or drug, etc., or using any techniques you can find that stop depression, it's also *very important* to "get a life"! In other words, to manage your life *more-skillfully*, so that you'll be happier and more successful. Often, the root cause of unhappiness is a mis-managed life! This author has also written another book, *Love*

Yourself: How to Actually Do It! This other book shows you how to create a happy life, full of more love, that needs no alcohol.

This mini-method #3 to stop alcohol, then, is really a method to *stop depression and unhappiness* (along with the need for better life-management).

Experiment to find what works best, for you, to stop unhappiness and depression. But, because unhappiness is also an *effect*, from the *cause* of a not-so-well-managed life, you'll eventually need to move to the *real cause* of unhappiness and manage your life more skillfully.

Anyway, it's all up to you to be *proactive* and do all this!

Mini-Method #4 - Diet

Eat sensibly, with foods and drinks that nourish your body! Avoid junk foods that just make your withdrawal symptoms worse. Also, avoid sweets, which at first give you a quick "sugar rush," but then lead to severe drops in blood sugar levels, later. A lower blood sugar level, when combined with withdrawal symptoms, will make it *much* harder not to drink more alcohol! Or, stop sugar (sucrose) altogether with Method #34.

Try not to eat more, after quitting alcohol. Fill up with more whole grains, fruits and vegetables. Try having small meals, but more frequently. Eat more protein, healthy fats (coconut oil, organic butter, fish) and non-starchy vegetables to give you more energy, that lasts! Eat a well-balanced diet, to give your body the 100 nutrients it needs every day. Eating eggs, yogurt, cheese, fish, and beans, in your meals and snacks, provides essential amino acids, probiotics, and healthy fats that will provide the energy and healthiness you need, to offset any withdrawal symptoms. *Organic foods* in your diet usually give you much more nutrition and fewer toxins, than non-organic foods, and are especially needed by your body at this time. Focus on eating the very healthiest, now!

Mini-Method #5 - Dream Quest of Unknown Kadath

H. P. Lovecraft once wrote an *incredible* short story entitled "The Dream Quest of the Unknown Kadath." The hero of this story, in a lucid dream state, searches for (and finds) the "realm of the gods," where he finally receives the answers that he seeks! Reading this amazing story may inspire you to try a similar quest yourself, for your "*stop alcohol*" *solutions*.

Is there any way, through *prayer*, *ritual*, *dance*, *ceremony*, or *contemplation/meditation*, that you could contact God, Jehovah, Allah, Buddha, Brahma, Jesus, Shiva, Vishnu, Great Spirit, or any other "Force-Of-God" that you know of or have heard of? How about a *god* from the culture of the Greeks, Romans, Norse, Hindus, Chinese, Japanese (Shinto), Egyptians (ancient), American Indians, Eskimos, or any other culture, with gods that you've read about or heard of? How about your Higher Self, your Angels, your Spiritual Guides, your Ancestors, or your Jungian archetypes (Self, Wise Old Man/Woman, Anima, Animus, Shadow, Trickster, Miraculous Child, Hero/Warrior/Savior), etc.

Anyway, try to *pick one of these* and then devise a way to get guidance on stopping alcohol, through *prayer*, *ritual*, *dance*, *ceremony*, or *contemplation/meditation*. Keep trying until you make it! Or you could even attempt, in a lucid dream or *lucid daydream*, to visit the "realm of the gods" to get your stop-alcohol solution, as they do in Eckankar (started by Paul Twitchell).

Mini-Method #6 - Hypnotherapy

This author's experience, in hypnotizing many people to stop alcohol, was that only 25% of people—who could go into a *deep* trance, actually stopped. The other 75%—who could only go into a *shallow* trance—didn't stop. However, none of my former hypnotic sessions included the extremely powerful "spittoon" technique, of Method #2, the "Hypnotic Extreme-Disgust Method." The success rate probably will increase to much more than 25% if the "spittoon" technique is used!

Also, if you use your own voice, or that of a trusted friend, it is more likely that you can relax into a *deep* trance.

If you go to a professional hypnotherapist, try to find one who's either inexpensive (in case it doesn't work), or one who will refund your money, if his/her hypnotherapy fails to stop alcohol use. Or, consider making your own self-hypnotic tape, to try.

Also, hypnosis can be combined with Mesmer's Animal Magnetism/*chi* (See Method #28, plus Method #29, too.)

Mini-Method #7 - Kudzu

Kudzu (Pueraria lobata), a Chinese herb, reduces alcohol cravings, to help drinkers to drink less. The extract *puerarin*, one of the isoflavones in kudzu, is one of the main ingredients causing this.

Drinking kudzu tea greatly discourages any alcohol consumption afterwards, by causing facial redness, nausea, and all-around discomfort (from any alcohol drunk after the kudzu tea).

Historically, in ancient China and Japan, kudzu tea was drunk to "sober up," more. Kudzu also is a remedy for alcoholic hangovers.

Kudzu in a tea seems to be significantly more effective than taking just the herb kudzu alone.

Mini-Method #8 - Managing Your Life Better

Directing, managing, or *wisely creating* your life seems essential to happiness and survival. Otherwise, the chaos, undone chores, and neglect of crucial responsibilities can serious undermine both happiness and survival! Of course, you can always "sort of get by," in living your life *randomly* (like a teenager). But the stress of unplanned living can be *exactly* what drives you to drink!

Make your own list of the 7, 10, or 12 important areas of life that *really matter* to you. This is my list:

(1) *Self-understanding*, of who you are are *at core*. Who are you really, deep down, and what do you *really* need to be doing, and how do you really need to be living your life, based on who this *deepest-core self* really is? If you already know (deeply) who you are, then take action! If you don't really know, get into meditation, psychology books, metaphysical books or seminars, or absolutely anything else (travel?) (asking best friends for feedback?) that works for you, here.

(2) *Health*. Create and start a nutritious diet and enjoyable, fun exercise program based on who you really are (deep down) and what you really like.

(3) *Money and Job.* If your job is "okay," keep doing it, I suppose. But if it's *beneath* the "okay" level, *eventually* attempt to change it. Usually not right away, because you need the money to live on! But start brainstorming what job you can switch to, even if it pays less and you need to be more-thrifty with the new, more-enjoyable job. In ten books I found on the internet, between them are listed over *3,000* entrepreneurial jobs, which you can start up on the side, with little money, until you can switch over from your regular job.

(4) *Relationship.* This is a tough, almost impossible one for me, I've found! Men and women have such different upbringings in American culture that they're practically *incompatible*! I've been in 47 romantic relationships with women, and all gradually deteriorated into quarreling, fighting, breaking up, and a broken heart. And almost everyone I've talked to or heard of goes through the same thing.

So, *get real*, here! Relationships *do* work at the beginning, when there's infatuation and a "honeymoon" phase going on. So, enjoy this "initially romantic" phase while it lasts (and watch your birth control), then end it *fast* when the verbal fighting begins! (Because the fighting will only get worse and worse until your heart is majorly broken, as you already know.)

Get good at writing personal ads for computer dating services. With skillful ads, at least you'll get 30-minute "blind dates," which can be interesting and educational. But, usually the rule of thumb here is that you can only get a partner of the same looks, age, and weight as yourself. So, if you want to find *better* romantic partners, you must improve *yourself*, in looks or weight. (Better clothes help, too.)

Finally, get a dog! (Or perhaps a cat?) After all, man's best friend is a dog (instead of a woman). Is it also true that woman's best friend is a *cat* (instead of a man)? (Occasionally, I hear people say, "I married my best friend," and these seem to be the only relationships that last.) Anyway, having a dog or cat really takes the *edge* off the loneliness of being single. And perhaps your pet will help you to drink less, if one of the predominant reasons you're drinking is loneliness for a relationship! Is this then the "Pet Cure" for those who over-drink? (We'll call this **Mini-Method #22 – Pet Cure**.)

(5) *Friends*. I've met most of these through the doing of fun hobbies. Join lots of clubs and go to social events that you like. Reach out and talk to others, and eventually you'll find some compatible friends. This often takes time and practice, but it's worth it in the end, especially if you're single!

(6) *Chores*. Try to find ways to make them more fun or enjoyable (like playing your favorite music) as you do them. Or, team up with a friend, to do both yours and his "most abominable" chores.

(7) *Fun and Hobbies*. Be sure to find time to fit these in, and they should be your *very favorite* hobbies (that you can comfortably afford).

Anyway, this is *my* list of seven life-goal-areas, to focus on. If you want to use this list of 7, fine. Or else, make up your own list. Your list should reflect who you truly are.

Finally, once *you* know who you are (deep down) and what you want out of life (your list of life-goal-areas), then *make it happen*! (And you'll probably cut down on the amount of alcohol you drink as you do this.)

Every day, plan your day, and do your plan, which is focused on being more-successful in your life-goal-areas. Of course, at first you'll very possibly succeed in being *only a little bit* better towards creating a better life, with more success in your life-goal areas. But, give yourself a break, and *appreciate* this little bit of success. Then, this self-appreciation of having "slightly more willpower" (in managing your life) will encourage you to do it a little bit more. And then a little bit more, still! Until, finally, you'll see a *significant improvement* in life-management ability! And it's this, the better, happier life that results from better life-management, that will work to *cut down on drinking alcohol*!

Conclusion: A better-managed life will greatly encourage you to *switch from booze* to the enthusiastic and joyous *living* of a happier and more-successful life!

Mini-Method #9 - Milk Thistle

Milk thistle (Silybum marianum) is an herbal remedy helping alcoholism, with the seeds called Shui Fei Ji in Chinese medicine. The silymarin in milk thistle helps cleanse alcohol and other poisons from the liver. Often nausea, abdominal pain, and loss of appetite result from alcohol-abuse liver disorders. Milk thistle was experimentally shown (by German scientists) to reduce all three of these symptoms!

Milk thistle helps the liver in many ways, when stopping alcohol, by preventing toxic chemicals from entering liver cells. Daily, take 420 mg (milligrams) of "silymarin" (standardized milk thistle extract), dividing into three doses, using a "standardized" milk thistle product.

Mini-Method #10 - Mindfulness Meditation

This helps soothe away the stress of alcohol withdrawal symptoms. Sit in a comfortable, quiet place, without distraction. Perhaps wear earplugs, to block out stressful noise. Perhaps wear green, color-therapy glasses, which are very restful and relaxing. Repeat a soothing "mantra" over and over (the mantra "I-YING, I-YING, I-YING", etc., works well), or "watch" (pay attention to) your breath (as in Vipassana meditation). Experiment with different meditations, to find out what works best, for you. Scientific books on mindfulness meditation have been written by Jon Kabat-Zinn, Ph.D., and Herbert Benson, M.D., if you would like to learn more why this method can be very helpful!

Rajneesh, or Osho, wrote about numerous good meditation techniques. Searching on the Internet can uncover at least a *dozen* different types of meditation, to experiment with.

Mini-Method #11 - Nutritional Supplements

Taking Vitamins A, B, C, D, and E replenishes a likely deficiency of them, caused by alcohol.

Also, Vitamins A, B, C, D, and E help in coping with alcohol withdrawal symptoms. A B-Vitamin capsule, pill, or powder (always keep B-Vitamins in your refrigerator!) that contains all eleven B-Vitamins, will help greatly.

A Multi-Mineral supplement (capsule, powder, or liquid) is good, too, and should include at least as much magnesium as calcium in it. Some people need twice as much magnesium as calcium, especially if you have "B" Blood Type. Some people need twice as much calcium as magnesium, but calcium is easier to get from food. A good Multi-Mineral supplement will also have chromium, selenium, and zinc, as well as trace minerals. Our body needs 100 nutrients daily, and about 60 of these are minerals! Natural Sea Salt has all of the minerals.

All of these vitamins and minerals will greatly help your health and energy, and will lessen the impact of alcohol withdrawal symptoms!

Mini-Method #12 - Passion Flower

This herb (Passiflora incarnata, or Passiflora quadrangularis) helps to calm, relax, and help relieve insomnia. It helps to reduce irritability and restlessness from alcohol withdrawal. It reduces alcohol cravings. For more information, you could check out this web page:

https://www.the-alcoholism-guide.org/herbal-treatment-for-alcoholism.html

Mini-Method #13 - Prosac

If you think that it's mainly *depression* that's causing your alcohol, then why not try *Prosac* (trade name for the prescription drug fluoxetine hydrochloride)? Numerous people are on Prosac these days, to stop depression.

Of course, St. John's wort (Method #14) is a better, healthier way to reduce or stop depression (and thus reduce or stop alcohol). Also, there are several other *herbs* (besides drugs) that reduce or stop depression. Try an internet search: "herbs that stop depression." Perhaps taking *several* "anti-depressant" herbs (all at once) would do the trick, here.

But if you don't want to bother with all this "herb stuff," then just take Prosac. Prosac may reduce or stop depression, which in turn will reduce or stop drinking alcohol.

Taking Prosac is a *lot* better for your health and your life than alcohol, by far!

But if you want to check it out for yourself, you can visit this website:

https://www.ehealthme.com/drug/prozac/side-effects/

Mini-Method #14 - Prosac-Alternative Prescription Drugs

Doctors and medical science are constantly coming up with new drugs that stop or reduce depression (to then stop or reduce alcohol use).

When you go into your doctor, to ask about Prosac, also ask about other antidepressant drugs that s/he might recommend.

Usually you have to *experiment* with new drugs to see if they *really do* stop your depression and alcohol). Also you need to find out if any unpleasant side-effects are caused.

By this experimentation, you might actually find *another* drug that works better than Prosac in stopping depression (and therefore alcohol).

Experimenting with various antidepressant *herbs* is possible too, and should cause fewer side-effects.

Starting out on Prosac (to stop depression and alcohol), but then later switching to other antidepressant drugs or anti-depressant herbs, is possible, too. Try it.

Mini-Method #15 - Skullcap Herb

Skullcap (Scutellaria lateriflora) helps to calm and heal the brain and nervous system, when you quit alcohol. It treats anxiety, nervousness, and insomnia. It reduces tension and stress. But, skullcap can also make you drowsy, so don't use it when alertness is needed. (Skullcap herb is also used in Method #10 - Dream Solution.)

Mini-Method #16 – Steam-Sweating Shower

When you quit alcohol, all the hundreds of toxins (from the alcohol) try to leave your body! This is one of the reasons why you feel so *miserable*, as the toxins go to your liver and kidneys, etc. Well, by sweating lots, in a hot shower, you can sweat a lot of the toxins out your skin, preventing them from going through your liver or kidneys!

Instructions for a Steam-Sweating Shower:

1) Cover your head with a towel dipped in cold water, and then squeezed out. It's a sort of "turban" you wear, to protect your brain from the extreme heat.

2) Take as hot a shower as your skin can possibly stand. As you do this, scrub your skin with a wash rag and a soap that absolutely *does not clog your skin's pores*! Don't use any soap with deodorant or additives or chemicals, which all clog your skin's pores, which reduces sweating! Recommended is either a natural soap or Ivory soap. Alternatively, using *Planet* brand *dishwashing liquid* is OK, because it will not clog pores and is certified to biodegrade to water, carbon dioxide, and healthful minerals.

3) Stand in the hot water shower, after washing off the soap, for about ten minutes, as you sweat and sweat and sweat! (It's possible for you to be sitting on a small stool here, instead of standing.) Have the hot water run down your back, as you stand or sit.

4) After ten minutes, turn the shower's water to *cold* (or as cold as you can stand it).

5) Scrub yourself off a second time, with the wash rag and soap, to remove all the oily sweat accumulated on the surface of your skin (that will harden, and feel terrible, if not scrubbed off in this second wash-rag scrubbing).

6) Step out of your "steam-sweating" shower, dry off, and feel how *good* your skin feels, and how much better *you* feel (from sweating out all those alcohol toxins and washing them away).

7) Drink plenty of water (filtered water is best), and eat some nourishing raw fruits or vegetables, to rebuild electrolyte and blood-nutrient levels (you may feel a little "tipsy", after all the sweating), and then some healthy protein and fats.

8) Don't drive your car for awhile, until you feel completely back to normal again, from eating healthy foods to rebuild nutrients that may have been sweated-out, along with the toxins.

Note: Do *not* do this steam-sweating shower if you have a *weak heart*! High water-temperatures in a shower, with a long session of sweating, can overly strain a weak heart.

Mini-Method #17 - Superfoods

There exist today several *superfoods*, plus vitamin and mineral supplements, which supply you with enormous amounts of nutritional energy!

Every day I eat plenty of:

(1) Raw Meal Protein Powder (5 heaping teaspoons)

(2) SunWarrior Protein Powder (2 heaping teaspoons)

(3) SunWarrior Super Greens (1 level teaspoon)

(4) Blue-green algae/spirulina/chlorella mix (1 level teaspoon)

(5) Reishi Mushroom (4 powder capsules)

(6) Cordyceps Mushroom (4 powder capsules)

(7) Vitamin A (25,000 IU)

(8) Vitamin B Complex (all eleven B vitamins in it) (1 capsule)

(9) Vitamin C (500 mg buffered with calcium and magnesium)

(10) Vitamin E (400 IU)

(11) Mega-Minerals (2 capsules)

All of these superfoods and supplements can be found on the internet and ordered.

I know this is quite a bit of supplements, but it makes me feel (physically) absolutely great! I also eat a nutritious, balanced diet, of mostly natural and organically grown foods, bought at a nearby health food store.

People abusing alcohol often have very poor nutrition! When nutrition is greatly improved, often alcohol craving tapers off, and significantly less alcohol is craved. There is a book by Joan Larson, PhD, called *Seven Weeks to Sobriety: The Proven Program to Fight Alcoholism through Nutrition* that goes into detail on this principle.

I greatly encourage anyone who is drinking too much alcohol to try a balanced, nutritional diet at some health food store in their vicinity, and to start taking all (or most) of the supplements that I've listed above.

Then, you'll feel nutritionally super too, and alcohol consumption should significantly decrease!

Mini-Method #18 - Support Network Creation

Include friends, and possibly family, to support your quitting. Perhaps even start a "Stop-Alcohol Support Network Group," with an ad on a bulletin board, on craigslist.org, Facebook, etc. Join up with special other people, who you can telephone, if you feel your resolve weakening. Find others who have quit! Then, try their method, with their support. "Quit-Alcohol Programs" can offer you extra support. Some of these are even free of charge. Ask around for them, or find them with an internet search.

Mini-Method #19 - Tablets of Zinc

Often those who drink a lot of alcohol are deficient in the trace mineral zinc. This is too bad, because zinc teams up with the liver, to reduce the toxicity of alcohol.

Taking zinc tablets regularly can help alcohol withdrawal symptoms. Also, zinc helps stop any brain dysfunction, or even seizures, that sometimes occur from reducing alcohol.

Alcohol cravings can lessen from taking zinc tablets regularly. Unfortunately, in our society there is widespread zinc deficiency, nowadays. This is despite the fact that zinc is quite an *essential nutrient*, needed to maintain good health!

50 mg to 80 mg every day, of zinc tablets, is the amount most health practitioners recommend. Try it, and see if you feel any of the above beneficial effects!

Mini-Method #20 - Vision Quest Method

Many American Indian tribes, for thousands of years, employed a traditional way to get answers to any serious question. It was to go on a so-called "Vision Quest."

Well, you can try this too, to get the answers you need, in your own unique way, on how *you* can stop drinking too much alcohol.

This technique is very powerful and often yields some very profound answers!

There are several ways to set in motion your Vision Quest. Because of this, I think it's best for you to do a search on the internet for all the various possible ways to do your Vision Quest. Then, you can decide which way feels best for you.

If one way of doing a Vision Quest doesn't fully work to your satisfaction, try a second way, or even a third way.

Good luck with this method. Its advantage is that your intuition, inner Muse, or Higher Self can point out to you what is the *absolute best way* for you to stop alcohol!

You can also try *lucid daydreaming* where, in a most daydreamy state, you gently direct the daydreamy inner world toward finding a stop-alcohol solution. Jung's "active imagination", or Eckankar, can be used here too. Jung repeatedly states that imagination is the source of all creative solutions.

Mini-Method #21 - Way of Random Choice

This is for those who can't make up their mind about which of the 34 methods and 23 mini-methods to try! All of these methods and mini-methods are just too overwhelming to some people! Well, instead of just throwing your hands in the air, in confusion and indecision, perhaps you could let a *card drawn at random* (from a deck of 52 playing cards plus Joker) decide which of the all the possibilities to try first. *Leave in the Joker(s)*!

INSTRUCTIONS

(1) From an ordinary deck of 52 playing cards plus Joker(s), draw *3 cards*, using all of your "intuitive powers," in carefully choosing these 3 cards!

(2) Match up your 3 cards to the list below, to arrive at 3 chosen Methods or Mini-Methods.

(3) Of the 3 choices, decide which one is to be your (favorite) Choice #1.

(4) Now you can

(a) only do your first choice, to stop your alcohol,

(b) combine your first choice with one of the other 2 choices, or

(c) combine your fist choice with *both* of the other 2 choices, so that you are using a "3-pronged attack" in your *campaign* to stop alcohol.

PLAYING CARDS PICKED, MATCHED UP WITH METHODS AND MINI-METHODS

Ace of Spades	Method #1: Gurdjieff-Inspired Method of Weaning
King of Spades	Method #2: Hypnotic Extreme-Disgust Method
Queen of Spades	Method #3: Self-Hypnosis to Take You to an Inner Guide
Jack of Spades	Method #4: The Banishing Alcohol Method
10 of Spades	Method #5: Quit in Three Months on Birthday Method
9 of Spades	Method #6: 6-A-Day Limit
8 of Spades	Method #7: Quit or Die
7 of Spades	Method #8: The Furious Anger Method
6 of Spades	Method #9: Affirm Quit Date
5 of Spades	Method #10: Dream Solution
4 of Spades	Method #11: Lucid Dreaming
3 of Spades	Method #12: Aerobic Shape
2 of Spades	Method #13: Strongest Muscles Press
Ace of Hearts	Method #14: St. John's Wort
King of Hearts	Method #15: Switch to Marijuana
Queen of Hearts	Method #16: Mixing "Lots of Fruity

	Drinks"
Jack of Hearts	Method #17: Passionate Hobby
10 of Hearts	Method #18: Why Do I Drink Method
9 of Hearts	Method #19: Reward Method
8 of Hearts	Method #20: Past-Life Ally Teamwork
7 of Hearts	Method #21: Subliminal Messages Method
6 of Hearts	Method #22: Near-Beer Guzzling
5 of Hearts	Method #23: Fake Booze While Smelling the Real
4 of Hearts	Method #24: Alternative Drug High
3 of Hearts	Method #25: Crying Out Sadness
2 of Hearts	Method #26: Brainwashing Yourself to Not Drink
Ace of Diamonds	Method #27: The Nine Nega-Emotions Method
King of Diamonds	Method #28: Mesmer's Animal Magnetism (not hypnosis)
Queen of Diamonds	Method #29: Ultra-Powerful Asiatic Hypnosis
Jack of Diamonds	Method #30: Magic Spell on Yourself
10 of Diamonds	Method #31: Role-Playing Parts A and B With a Friend (in last two paragraphs of Method #30)
9 of Diamonds	Method #32: Put Together Your Own Method (from other bits and pieces of this book)
8 of Diamonds	Method #33: Love Yourself Method

7 of Diamonds	Method #34: Stopping Sugar
6 of Diamonds	Mini-Method #1: Ally-Archetype Sub-Self Method
5 of Diamonds	Mini-Method #2: Cayenne Pepper
4 of Diamonds	Mini-Method #3: Depression Stopping Method
3 of Diamonds	Mini-Method #4: Diet
2 of Diamonds	Mini-Method #5: Dream Quest of Unknown Kadath
Ace of Clubs	Mini-Method #6: Hypnotherapy
King of Clubs	Mini-Method #7: Kudzu
Queen of Clubs	Mini-Method #8: Managing Your Life Better
Jack of Clubs	Mini-Method #9: Milk Thistle
10 of Clubs	Mini-Method #10: Mindfulness Meditation
9 of Clubs	Mini-Method #11: Nutritional Supplements
8 of Clubs	Mini-Method #12: Passion Flower
7 of Clubs	Mini-Method #13: Prosac
6 of Clubs	Mini-Method #14: Prosac Alternative Drugs
5 of Clubs	Mini-Method #15: Skullcap
4 of Clubs	Mini-Method #16: Steam Sweat
3 of Clubs	Mini-Method #17: Superfoods
2 of Clubs	Mini-Method #18: Support Network
JOKER	Mini-Method #19: Tablets of Zinc

JOKER	Mini-Method #20: Vision Quest
JOKER	Mini-Method #22: Pet Cure (in paragraph 4 of Mini-Method #8: Managing Your Life Better), or
JOKER	Mini-Method #23: Reichian Therapy

Table 1. Linking playing cards with Methods and Mini-Methods

Of course, most rational, logical, scientifically minded people would say that one should choose one of the 34 Methods or 23 Mini-Methods by:

(1) analysis and logic, or

(2) emotional appeal, or

(3) practicality and common sense.

But, who knows? Perhaps choosing by this "Way of Random Choice" might be equally effective! Consider trying it!

Obviously, it's not "either-or" here. Thus, choice of method or mini-method can *primarily* be by your usual, personality-based way of deciding things. Then a *secondary* choice can be made by this "Way of Random Choice" method. And then perhaps your *primary choice*, and your *secondary choice*, can be combined?

Anyway, your use of this "Way of Random Choice" mini-method is (obviously) completely up to you. In fact, instead of using the card deck, you can apply a "dowsing rod" to the Table of Contents to choose. Your "dowsing rod" can perhaps be made from a paper clip, or from 2 pens taped together at their ends.

Good luck!

Mini-Method #22 - Pet Cure

(See Mini-Method #8.)

Mini-Method #23 - Reichian Therapy

This is especially for those who are *really blocked* from crying and "can't cry" anymore.

HOW TO DO IT:

Lie down on a bed, face up. Bend your knees, so that your knees are pointed at the ceiling (as you lie there on the bed). Now, start a deep breathing process. Inhale and exhale strongly, over and over. This hyperventilation should start to make you feel your repressed anger, sadness, and fear, etc. Allow yourself to *feel* all this, as you pound the mattress with your fists coming down onto the mattress on either side of your body, intensely. (Don't injury your hands, here.) Allow the repressed emotions that have been locked up inside you to *explode*, like a volcano! Shout, yell, cry, or make any other (unusual) sounds that need to emerge from your throat. Keep at it, until you've had a big release, and the process gradually "peters out," until you're relaxed again, having discharged a whole chunk of pent-up emotion that was festering deeply inside yourself. For, all this buried emotion may have been what was driving you to *drink*. So, it greatly needs to be released!

Caution (1): The noise you make could likely alarm the neighbors! So you might have to drive your car to a deserted area and do it in the car, where nobody can hear you. (Don't get mugged in a deserted area of town.) This author has learned to *relax his vocal chords*, as he does this process, so that all that is heard is a bunch of (relatively silent) *air* being forcefully breathed out, over and over.

Caution (2): This process can easily *open an emotional door* between your conscious and subconscious! This door, once opened, could stay open for a few days or even a week! Thus, your conscious mind could be flooded with this backlog of volatile repressed emotions for days or a week afterward. And there may not be a "shut-off lever" or "button," to stop it! Thus, your work and your life may be severely compromised for a few days (or a week) afterward, by *tidal waves* of repressed emotion emerging from your subconscious, to blast your conscious mind. Perhaps you could have a friend with you, during the Reichian Therapy process, to start yelling at you to stop after, say, five minutes. This friend may need to even grab your shirt and start to shake you, as he yells, "Stop! It's been 5 minutes already! Stop, stop, stop!" This way, with only 5 minutes of release, perhaps the repression barrier in your mind will *stay* intact, to stop the "leakage" of intense buried emotion into *your* conscious mind afterwards for hours, days, or even a week.

You may consider going to a professional Reichian Therapist (although it's expensive). Or, you may put an ad on craigslist.org, asking advice from someone who has tried Reichian Therapy to explain it to you, and *especially* explain how he eventually learned to conduct his *own* free *solo-sessions* without danger.

Or, you could try your first session at the beginning of a week-long vacation from work.

Or, you could attempt an initial solo-session of Reichian Therapy at 6 p.m. on a Friday, right after your 5-day workweek. Then you'll have 2-1/2 days to emotionally recover before Monday morning. This plan would work even better if you have the option of calling in sick on Monday, or even Tuesday, too. But if this "Reichian at 6 PM Friday" plan works, with a weekend offering any emotional recovery needed, then perhaps doing *regular* Reichian solo-sessions every week, or even every *two* weeks, will release enough pent-up, repressed, negative energy for you to significantly cut down on drinking alcohol, or *even stop*!

An alternative to Reichian sessions is to get a steel-frame tennis racket and a cloth-filled sack of dry rice. "Whack the shit" out of the rice sack with the tennis racket, as you yell out your pent-up emotions. When most of your rage has been "whacked out," you could try lying on your right side (on the rug) and crying. Then after the crying peters out, force yourself to *laugh*, as uproariously as possible, at the cosmic absurdity of it all! Then another cycle of "Pound-Cry-Laugh," etc. Beginners at this should stop after just *one* cycle, then wait several hours to see how much "flooding" of emotion from the subconscious occurs.

It's also possible to "kick the shit" out of a bunch of cardboard boxes in your backyard, as you either yell, or relax your vocal chords, so that only a lot of "air" sound is heard.

Good luck here, with all of these rage-release techniques, and crying! They really work to release the core emotions that trigger you to drink!

AFTERWORD

MORE METHODS NEEDED! PLEASE!

I believe that the best way, to help people to stop alcohol, is to provide them with *lots and lots* of methods that actually work! Then, people can choose the method that works for them, *do* this method, and stop!

If you know of *any* other method to stop alcohol, *please* let me know of it! Or, if you tried a *combination* of methods in this book that worked, then email *that combination* to me. Send to my email: garypickler1@gmail.com (don't forget the "1" after my name). Thank you!

When I receive enough methods from you and others, I will write a second book, *More Methods To Stop Alcohol Fast!*, and all contributors will get a free copy.

Let's get these "stop alcohol methods" out into the world, as fast as we can, to help all those with alcohol issues who are trapped in their alcohol addiction!

Also, if you liked this book, *please* give it a 5-star review, to encourage others to get it and let it work for them, too! Thank you, thank you, so much!

Let's help as many people as we can to more-effectively deal with their alcohol issues, to heal and change their lives for the better, to enable them to start living the happy, successful, cured-from-alcohol life that they've always wanted, deep down in their souls!

www.ingramcontent.com/pod-product-compliance
Lightning Source LLC
Chambersburg PA
CBHW051427280526
45785CB00003B/1197